# 12-Step Zen

## Pathways of Recovery

Peter Kuhn



Parallax Press

Berkeley, California

Parallax Press
PO Box 7355
Berkeley, CA 94707
parallax.org

Parallax Press is the publishing division of Plum Village Community of Engaged Buddhism, Inc.



Thich Nhat Hanh's poems "Unclasp" on page x and "Walking Meditation" on page 116 are from *Call Me by My True Names: The Collected Poems of Thich Nhat Hanh*, courtesy of the publisher.
"And When I Rise" on page 106 is from *Basket of Plums Songbook*, courtesy of the publisher.
"Enter Your Life" by Dr. Larry Ward on page 128 is from *Morning Night*, by permission of Lotus Moss Press.

Cover design by Katie Eberle
Cover art by Lily Kong
Text design by Maureen Forys, Happenstance Type-O-Rama
Author photograph by Kevin Tevares
Images on pages 58, 92, 124, and 147 courtesy of Plum Village

Printed on FSC-certified paper in the United States of America by Versa

Parallax Press's authorized representative in the EU and the EEA is SAS Plum Village at Home—Point UH, 437 Chemin du Pey, Thénac, France | Email: europe@parallax.org

Library of Congress Cataloging-in-Publication Data
Names: Kuhn, Peter (Addiction recovery advocate) author
Title: 12-step Zen : pathways of recovery / Peter Kuhn.
Other titles: Twelve-step Zen
Description: Berkeley, California : Parallax Press, [2026] | Summary: "An unflinching and compassionate exploration of addiction, healing, and renewal through Zen practice and Twelve-Step recovery"—Provided by publisher.
Identifiers: LCCN 2026027985 (print) | LCCN 2026027986 (ebook) | ISBN 9781888375695 trade paperback | ISBN 9781888375855 ebook
Subjects: LCSH: Substance abuse—Alternative treatment | Twelve-step programs | Substance abuse—Religious aspects—Buddhism | Twelve-step programs—Religious aspects—Buddhism | Zen Buddhism | LCGFT: Popular works
Classification: LCC RC564.29 .K78 2026 (print) | LCC RC564.29 (ebook)
LC record available at https://lccn.loc.gov/2026027985
LC ebook record available at https://lccn.loc.gov/2026027986

1 2 3 4 5 VERSA 30 29 28 27 26

MIX
Paper | Supporting responsible forestry
FSC® C005010
FSC www.fsc.org

# PRAISE FOR *12-STEP ZEN*

"Weaving together the Buddha's teachings, the Twelve Steps, and his musical background, Peter Kuhn shares his poignant healing journey through trauma and addiction—offering deep insight and meaningful support to those of us and families navigating various forms of addiction as we find our way back to ourselves and build more fulfilling lives."

—**SISTER DANG NGHIEM**, MD, author of *Live Beautifully, Die Beautifully*

"The book that you hold in your hands is a treasure born from the lived experience and insight of one of the most compassionate people I am lucky to know. Skillfully weaving together personal stories, actionable insights, and concrete practices, *12-Step Zen* is an essential resource for all practitioners, and I am deeply grateful that this book is now available. I know that I will be returning to it over and over again. I can't recommend it highly enough."

—**BROTHER PHÁP HAI**, author of *The Eight Realizations of Great Beings*

"With this profound book, Peter Kuhn takes us from the depths of addiction and its concomitant miseries to a clear-eyed and measured awakening to what he refers to as *12-Step Zen*. It's a journey that so many addicts rarely survive, let alone find leading them to a profound teacher, a caring community, and lasting sobriety. Thank you, Peter, for this luminous gift."

—**NELS CLINE**, composer and guitarist (Wilco)

"*12-Step Zen* offers apt medicine for our suffering. Taste and see!"

—**GARY GACH**, author of *The Complete Idiot's Guide to Buddhism* and *Pause, Breathe, Smile: Awakening Mindfulness When Meditation Is Not Enough*

"Peter Kuhn offers a heartfelt guide to the changes that lead to true health and happiness. This practice flows deep in his blood and abides in his essence. I have personally witnessed him touch thousands of lives, and this book will undoubtedly continue that inspiring work."

—**JEFF ZLOTNIK**, cofounder of the Dharma Bum Temple

"Written with a musician's sensitivity and the inward clarity of one shaped by recovery, Peter Kuhn's deeply felt book brings the wisdom of Twelve-Step practice into rich and searching dialogue with Buddhism's Seven Factors of Awakening. This is a work shaped by lived experience—by loss and longing, by addiction and grace, and by the redemptive discipline of meditation. This is a book about recovery, yes—but beneath it all runs the deeper music of awakening."

—**THÉRÈSE JACOBS-STEWART,** author of *Mindfulness and the 12 Steps*

"Peter Kuhn uses the ancient and timeless teachings of the Buddha as well as modern Twelve-Step wisdom as wonderful guides for release from suffering. The most inspiring part of this book for me is the fearless, transparent sharing of his own journey. Kuhn makes what could be overwhelming topics easy to access, put in the context of his very interesting life."

—**ROSHI ANNE SEISEN SAUNDERS,** Abbot Emeritus, Sweetwater Zen Center

"*12-Step Zen* is a deeply honest and compassionate exploration of recovery, awakening, and the freedom that becomes possible when mindfulness and the Twelve Steps truly come alive together. Peter Kuhn writes with the wisdom of lived experience, offering a path that transforms suffering into clarity, resilience, and an open-hearted way of being."

—**JOHN BRUNA,** cofounder of the Mindfulness in Recovery® Institute, spiritual director of the Way of Compassion Dharma Center, and author of *The Essential Guidebook to Mindfulness in Recovery*

"Two seemingly disparate wisdom traditions in this book have been woven together in a unique and enormously helpful way: the Twelve-Step tradition and the Buddhist teaching of the Seven Factors of Enlightenment. Both paths start out with the acknowledgment of suffering and its causes and end with tools that, if followed rigorously and grounded in mindfulness, will not only reduce suffering greatly but also encourage compassion and joy. But what really animates this book is Peter Kuhn's own personal path from addiction to non-attachment and his experiential interface with both traditions. *12-Step Zen* is a major text for those seeking to understand what addiction and recovery truly look like."

— **RICHARD AVERY,** LCSW, Certified Compassion Cultivation Trainer, Vipassana teacher, psychotherapist, and assistant professor, UCSD Department of Psychiatry

*To my teacher, Thich Nhat Hanh,*
*and to all my spiritual ancestors*
*in Twelve-Step recovery and the*
*noble Buddhist lineage*

# CONTENTS

## PART III
## The Refuge Dwells in Me

## UNCLASP

*Deserted beach,*
*footsteps in the sand*
*erased by rain—*
*this anguish comes from nowhere,*
*and its feet do not yet touch the Earth.*
*Suddenly I hear a far-off whisper*
*of the gentle winds of spring,*
*and the anguish is gone.*

–THICH NHAT HANH

# FOREWORD

The great Vietnamese Zen master Thich Nhat Hanh understood suffering. He watched his beloved homeland ravaged by the devastating violence of the American military, and yet, out of that horrific experience, he developed a heart of boundless compassion. There's no doubt that Thay (as he was known to his students) would have responded in the same way to Peter Kuhn's account of addiction, recovery, and immersion in the Dharma.

These pages take us through the harrowing journey of a hope-to-die junkie and his remarkable escape to freedom. Kuhn, now a full-fledged Dharma teacher himself, displays a wisdom and understanding of the great teachings of the Buddha. His ability to translate these for other recovering addicts is a gift to be savored. Using the framework of the Seven Factors of Awakening, he skillfully guides us through the flowering of wisdom that the Buddha promises. For anyone seeking a way to deepen recovery and find joy and meaning in this very life, this will be a treasured guidebook.

Kuhn is part of a larger movement in the recovery world to integrate Buddhism in our healing. While Twelve-Step and other programs continue to have tremendous value in dealing with these pernicious addictive conditions, this century has seen the growth of something new, what's called "Buddhist recovery." This path offers a non-theistic, contemplative approach to these age-old problems. The practice of mindfulness and the wisdom inherent to the Buddhist tradition allow for an intimacy with pain, create space for self-examination, and ultimately make possible a peace that so often proves elusive, even for someone in recovery. *12-Step Zen* is an invaluable contribution to this growing movement.

—**KEVIN GRIFFIN,** author of *One Breath at a Time: Buddhism and the Twelve Steps* and other books

# PRELUDE

I love music, and for years, it was my passion and reason for living. It was a refuge and identity that allowed me to express my spirit and did not interfere with my drug use. I considered drugs as medicine, and in the early years, narcotics gave me a semblance of spiritual peace. They helped me settle and focus enough to practice four to six hours a day. In live performance, they helped quiet the running thoughts that relentlessly fed my doubts and insecurities. When I was high, I was in the groove, I felt more in the moment and at one with the music. My improvisations flowed on what felt like a tide of pure spirit. Many of my music heroes had been drug addicts, and I thought addiction was an acceptable part of that life. Music was a lifeline until addiction brought me to the edge of ruin and, eventually, to recovery.

In the mid-1970s, when I was in my early twenties, I moved to New York City, which was considered the jazz capital of the world. The music scene was flourishing there, and I hoped to make my mark. Drugs were plentiful, and I was in a community of world-class players. I released my first album, *Livin' Right*, two years after arriving, and it helped me to convince myself that I really had it going on. The album featured original compositions, and the press was favorable.

I thought I was doing everything right, but the conditions I had created were unsustainable. I had the trappings of success, but I was spiritually empty. I hid behind the musician's persona to justify my lonely, lost, and inadequate existence. If someone asked how I was doing, I just told them about a gig, recording, or review, which were the trappings of success.

Not everyone in the jazz scene used drugs. For some, music was a path of spiritual awakening. John Coltrane, one of the great jazz masters, kicked his habit in the '60s and became a role model of spiritual living and freedom in music. By the time I moved to New York City, I realized being an addict was no longer hip, but I felt like I needed it to be creative and survive. I was truly convinced that God put narcotics on the planet so I could function on a higher level.

I thought of addiction as a victimless pursuit, even as I committed crimes to support my habit. I believed in peace and love, but ethical conduct wasn't on my map. My mind was cloudy, but I rationalized that I was just a dreamer—my contribution to the world was my music, and if even one person felt good listening to it, I was successful. If I got sick at times, arrested, and desperate, I shrugged it off as a small part of the life I had chosen for myself.

Some jazz elders in the city, responsible and socially conscious, opened performance spaces called lofts to serve the community of creative, noncommercial jazz artists. The loft era was a cultural phenomenon, and I was fortunate to be there during that time.

Ali's Alley was owned and operated by Rashied Ali, who had played with John Coltrane during the final years of Coltrane's life. He even had a liquor license. I remember sitting at his bar shortly after the release of *Livin' Right* and telling him about it, full of pride and a little boastful. I couldn't see that I was what Buddhists call a hungry ghost—endlessly seeking praise, approval, and relief from the outside.* High on drugs and good press, I hoped to impress Rashied, maybe get a gig at his legendary club.

He met my eyes across the bar and asked softly, "Are you living right, Peter?"

I didn't recognize it as old-style schooling or appreciate the gift Rashied was offering. I was taken aback that he saw right through me. I bluffed and blustered to cover the cold dread of shame that washed over me. Playing it off, I said something like, "Hell yeah, I sure think so." Rashied looked at me kindly and shrugged before

---

* In Buddhist teachings, a hungry ghost is a being tormented by insatiable craving and endless dissatisfaction. They are traditionally depicted with enormous empty bellies, a pencil-thin neck, and a small mouth.

turning his back to polish a glass or dust a bottle. I mumbled a few words as I finished my drink and made a hasty exit for the safety of the street.

In 1982, I was twenty-eight and coming out of a romantic breakup. My emotional range was limited to a few states. If I had money to get well in the morning and the dope was good, I was happy. Otherwise, I was mad, sad, or sick.

I was invited to tour Europe with the Original Bass Clarinet Choir and hoped the music and a change of scenery might ease the pain in my heart. On the outside, things were great, and my musical dreams were coming true.

But the oppressive weight of loneliness and loss came with me. The music brought moments of relief, times when I lost myself in the resonant sound of the bass clarinets. Sadness flowed through me like a slow river of blues.

Our tour ended in an acoustically superb concert hall in Salzburg, Austria, before the largest audience of the trip. It was my last hurrah with the group, and I poured myself into the music. Afterward, an excited press corps came backstage to sing our praises. One writer said he could hear the influence of Eric Dolphy and John Coltrane in my playing, high praise indeed. But in that moment of accomplishment when I might have rejoiced, I felt hollow.

In the years that followed, I tried to clean up many times. I knew I needed to stop but didn't know how. When I wasn't on drugs, my life felt like a swamp of suffering. Four more years passed before the pain I tried to avoid brought me to my knees and revealed a door to freedom. I finally got clean on January 5, 1986.

I later learned a simple truth: the way out is in. In my music and recovery, I find harmony in the dissonance of my human experience. This became my path of Zen recovery.

# INTRODUCTION
# The Weave Beneath the Words

In traditional jazz, a song has a melody and an underlying harmonic structure, the chord changes, that provide the ground for improvisation. Our lives may seem well composed, yet each day we make countless choices: what to eat, what to say, how to respond to a given situation. Our lives are living music, and each of us is an improvising artist. As we develop our craft, we discover that moments of happiness are possible even in a world that includes discomfort and sorrow.

As a recovering addict, I have navigated highs and lows for more than forty years. The freedom and joy I have experienced surpass anything intoxicants ever offered. The hardships and challenges have been equally profound. With the tools of recovery, I learned to meet them as opportunities rather than obstacles, though the path has not always been easy.

After a devastating death in 2002, when I had sixteen years clean, I encountered Zen through the teachings of Thich Nhat Hanh. It changed the trajectory of my life. In the decades since, the Twelve-Step and Buddhist paths have come to breathe together, helping me find harmony in a lifetime of struggle and dissonance. I explore this journey in the pages that follow.

This book is built on the harmonic framework of the Seven Factors of Awakening, which are ordinary capacities of the mind that can be cultivated. Through that framework run the melodic lines of the Twelve Steps and the living tradition of Plum Village Zen. My hope is to offer a primer on both wisdom streams—a song for you to play and develop in your own beautiful way.

True freedom is the growing capacity to be at ease with unease. It is the ability to feel our feelings fully, without being overwhelmed, and to live with dignity as the sovereign of our own lives. No longer driven by craving or governed by fear, we find the spaciousness to inhabit our lives with open hearts: present, awake, and responsive to life as it unfolds. Sometimes it's as simple as staying present during an argument instead of storming out. It is the freedom offered by both recovery and the Buddhist teachings, the capacity to be fully alive, right here, right now.

Living mindfully in recovery, I've learned to nourish happiness and transform suffering with kindness and care. We all have this capacity. We are not victims. When I use words like addiction and recovery, I'm pointing toward what the Buddha described as suffering and the end of suffering. Suffering includes any form of discomfort, unhappiness, or affliction.

For an addict, freedom often begins by asking for help and abstinence. For you, it may begin elsewhere.

The Twelve Steps have been adapted and applied in hundreds of anonymous fellowships that address a wide range of struggles, from money and food to grief and trauma. In the same spirit, I trust that readers familiar with recovery and those new to it may find value in these principles, just as many have benefited from the Buddha's teachings.

Twelve-Step literature describes addiction as a spiritual malady. Abstinence from intoxicants is a prerequisite for the awakening promised in the Twelfth Step. In Buddhist practice, refraining from intoxicants is one of the Five Precepts the Buddha offered.* Abstinence clears the ground. It is not an end in itself but a condition that makes clarity and freedom possible. As we move through the

* The Five Precepts are (1) not killing, (2) not stealing, (3) avoiding sexual misconduct, (4) refraining from false speech, and (5) abstaining from intoxicants.

Steps, what begins as abstinence deepens into a way of life guided by spiritual principles.

We learn to recognize and refrain from unskillful patterns of thought, speech, and action. As we live the program, abstinence naturally expands into the ethical awareness expressed in the other precepts.

The intersection of Twelve-Step recovery and Buddhist wisdom remains endlessly rich and alive for me. These two streams inform and enliven one another. My connection with both communities sustains my well-being and keeps my understanding fresh and evolving.

Problems are inevitable. What matters is how we engage with them. The Twelve Steps offer one path. Zen Master Thich Nhat Hanh spoke of both the art of living and the art of suffering. As he put it, "The art of happiness is at the same time the art of suffering well. When we learn to suffer, we suffer much, much less."* As a jazz musician, I think of this art as improvisation on an ever-shifting set of dynamics and changes.

The Twelve Steps and the Seven Factors appear throughout this book, but not in even measure or tidy sequence. Recovery and awakening don't unfold that way. As a musician, I learned that what matters most is not keeping time perfectly, but learning when to listen, when to respond, and when to let a phrase resolve in its own way. We return to certain steps again and again, while others recede for long stretches. Some practices arrive early; others only make sense later. I invite you to read this book the way recovery unfolds, as a living, unmetered practice guided by attention rather than consumption.

The Buddha taught in an oral tradition, and many of his teachings, like the Four Noble Truths and the Noble Eightfold Path, were numbered to help people remember. If numbered lists feel

---

* Thich Nhat Hanh, *No Mud, No Lotus: The Art of Transforming Suffering* (Parallax Press, 2014), 3.

off-putting, don't worry. No memorization is required. I hope you'll look to the substance and hear the music beneath the words; the living practice they point toward.

When I first attended meetings, I heard the adage, "Take what you can use and file the rest away for future reference." Not everything we hear or read is immediately understood or useful. Some of the teachings in this book were confusing when I first encountered them. Others eluded me for years.

Developing a working understanding of the Steps and Buddhist teachings takes time, repeated exposure, and reflection. I've tried to make this book accessible while including deeper material that adds some complexity to the weave. I share these because they have been meaningful to me, and I hope they will be of value to you. In a culture of soundbites, I encourage you to take your time with them, as a gift to yourself that in turn will benefit all beings.

If you are suffering from active addiction or other afflictions, please don't doubt your capacity to heal and transform. No matter the harm we've caused or how hopeless things may feel, we are all worthy of love and support. Help is available. Paths to freedom can help us harmonize our lives, discover meaning, and awaken the song in our hearts. I hope this book illuminates one such path.

May we walk it together.

# PART I

# Taking Refuge: There Is a Path

THE FIRST FACTOR OF AWAKENING:

# Mindfulness

## Waking Up to Life

What is mindfulness? That depends on who you ask. The word and the practices it encompasses mean different things to different people. In sleek corporate offices, mindfulness has become the latest productivity hack, another strategy for getting more done. Athletes use it to sharpen their competitive edge, to find the zone where performance peaks. The military employs it to help soldiers stay focused and steady amid chaos and peril. In hospitals and clinics, it's offered to help with chronic pain and depression and to ease stress and anxiety. It's been adapted for sleep therapy, helping people rest when their minds won't quiet. And for those of us in recovery, mindfulness-based relapse prevention helps us recognize and pause when old patterns begin to call us back. In all these settings, mindfulness appears as a practical tool with proven results.

A friend once told me he practices mindfulness while watching television, because he's "in the moment," completely absorbed in the show. The word has been so widely co-opted that there's even a television series called *Murder Mindfully*.

Buddhist mindfulness is rooted in a 2,500-year-old wisdom tradition. It can be used for stress reduction or performance, but its deeper aim is transformation. It is a path of remembrance and discovery that transforms suffering and nurtures the freedom and well-being that are our birthright.

Mindfulness, as the Buddha taught it, is being compassionately awake to life as it unfolds: meeting each moment with openhearted attention and a spirit of goodwill toward ourselves and what we encounter. It invites us to wake up to the truth of our lives, moment by moment, with gentleness, curiosity, and care. Rooted in ethical living and nourished by compassion, Buddhist mindfulness invites us to touch the freedom, clarity, and well-being that are already here, already present within us.

In that steady awareness, we begin to see clearly and transform our relationship to suffering. Touching our pain with tenderness, we discover our Buddha nature—the mind of love. It is our "recovery nature."

Mindfulness is the beating heart of the Buddha's teachings; it is a factor of awakening, integral to the Noble Eightfold Path of liberation.*

Some people see recovery programs as a means to an end, simply a way to stop drinking or using. Abstinence is a doorway, not the destination. In recovery, we learn to live in the world as it is, with serenity. The program is a path of discovery and transformation. The Steps help us understand the causes of suffering and point to a spiritual solution.

Both wisdom paths guide us to care for suffering and nourish happiness. It's easy to get on board with nourishing happiness. I thought I was doing that with drugs. But who wants to care for suffering, to face unavoidable pain? For a long time, my answer was to deny or defy the fears, hurts, and problems that seemed like a plague sent to prove my unworthiness. The Buddha called suffering a noble truth. What does that mean, and how could suffering possibly be noble?

---

* The Noble Eightfold Path is to practice Right View, Right Intention, Right Speech, Right Action, Right Livelihood, Right Effort, Right Concentration, and Right Mindfulness.

## Is Suffering Noble?

I started getting high at ten, and trouble quickly followed. By my early teens, I had been arrested and busted for drugs at two schools. After being expelled from the second, I entered my first long-term rehabilitation program in 1968. I was fourteen.

There weren't many treatment centers in those days. This one was called Synanon, and at first, it was exciting. I was out of school, away from my parents, living in a community of addicts, alcoholics, and criminals. I regarded them as wise elders. I didn't want to stop using; it was like a trade school in advanced addiction.

I met fascinating characters and learned confidence games, crimes, and hustles. I was also exposed to great jazz and musicians like Art Pepper, who mentioned meeting me there in his autobiography, *Straight Life*. People encouraged me to read widely—writers such as Ralph Waldo Emerson and Henry David Thoreau—and introduced me to the work of R. Buckminster Fuller, a visionary inventor and philosopher.

After fifteen months at Synanon, I returned to public school and met Fuller's grandson, Jamie. He introduced me to "Bucky," and I sought out opportunities to spend time with him whenever he came to town. He drank tea all day—something I now do as well—and I kept his teapot full, ran errands, and listened deeply. He saw himself as a generalist rather than a specialist, describing his work as "comprehensive anticipatory design science." He helped me learn to see patterns.

Bucky told me he had once been an alcoholic and, with a wife and young child, had fallen into suicidal depression. As he contemplated taking his life, he wondered whether there was any meaning or purpose to it all. Instead of acting, he decided to take a year to reflect and made a vow of silence during that time.

In a moment of clarity, he concluded that since we all have problems, our purpose must be problem-solving.

He intuitively arrived at two aspects of the Noble Eightfold Path: Right View and Right Mindfulness. "Right" is sometimes translated as "wise," pointing toward well-being and freedom from suffering rather than moral judgment. Right Mindfulness is asking a simple question: What are we paying attention to, and where is it leading us? Right View is recognizing that problems can reveal solutions. Problems and solutions define each other. The pairs of opposites we experience in life arise together and depend on one another.

One day, when I was hanging out with Bucky, I tried to impress him with a scathing commentary I'd borrowed from my older brother. I was fishing for praise, but he said, "Peter, it's easy to be brilliantly negative. The challenge is to be brilliantly positive and find solutions to our problems."

The wisdom of that guidance still resonates with me, both in the Dharma (Buddhist teachings) and in recovery. The Buddha taught a simple arc, referred to as the Four Noble Truths: we suffer; suffering has causes; freedom is possible; and there is a path. Though the Buddha taught about suffering, his teaching points toward the cessation of suffering—brilliantly positive in its aim. When I heard the Twelve-Step program described as "solution-oriented" many years after this conversation with Bucky and my first encounters with mindfulness, I felt a quiet sense of recognition and alignment. Thanks to Bucky, I trusted that these ways of being free were possible.

As Bucky concluded, problems are an opportunity for problem-solving. Suffering—the first of the Four Noble Truths—is not a wall but a Dharma door. It is an invitation, not a destination. With Right View and Right Mindfulness, pain and suffering can become a friendly warning system. They point us to the causes of suffering and reveal the possibility of freedom.

We all want to be happy. The pursuit of happiness is even named as an unalienable right in the United States Declaration of Independence. Drugs were my idea of happiness. But what happens when our idea of happiness becomes the very cause of our suffering?

## Samsara: The Cycle of Suffering

I thought of drugs as emotional alchemy. They magically changed my mood and how I felt about you, me, and my life. Sure, they caused problems, but I chalked those up to bad luck and circumstance.

Drugs were my medicine, friend, and lover. They got me out of bed in the morning and helped me sleep at night. Incarceration, sickness, and eventual homelessness were simply the price to pay. A fair trade, I thought—until it became too much to bear.

Everything that disturbed me seemed a curse, proof of my unworthiness and the unfairness of life. In the end, I looked and smelled like an addict. People would literally cross the street to avoid me. I needed to stop, but abstinence felt like a loss. I couldn't let go of the idea that drugs had something to offer me.

I left New York City in 1981, hoping I could clean up in Los Angeles. That didn't work out. In 1985, I was released from LA County Jail for the last time and took a bus to Santa Monica, where I had left my car, a Ford Pinto. The ocean air felt good and smelled fresh. I had nowhere to go, but I tried to put a spring in my step. Everything would be different this time. I would get a girlfriend and a job and stay away from narcotics.

As I walked up to the friend's house where my car waited, I was a man with a plan. I could hear the TV inside and stopped to take a breath. I was clear about my plan: I was not going to use heroin. This was a new beginning.

I was shocked when I opened the screen door. Trash was piled in the corner. I could smell the mountain of garbage in the kitchen, and the living room looked like a tornado had hit it. My cell was cleaner than this. My friend Freddie was slouched in an old armchair in front of a small black-and-white TV sitting on a milk crate with a coat-hanger antenna.

Freddie was obviously loaded—his eyes drooped, and his chin rested on his chest. A lit cigarette dangled from his hand, the ash two inches long. As I stood in the doorway, I was surprised by my first thought: I wondered if he had more. Absurd as it sounds, his inebriated state looked good to me. It was an out-of-body experience watching myself ask for drugs. My gut was telling me no, but the pull of desire overpowered it. Fuck it. I'd been locked up. I had a high coming. The thought of getting high became an obsession. Where was mine?

I was defenseless. My plans went out the window. I was off and running again.

They say insanity is doing the same thing over and over and expecting different results. Buddhists call this cycle of repeated suffering the wheel of *samsara*: the endless loop of wanting, getting, regretting, repeating. Did I expect things to be different this time? In the grip of obsession, the question never arose. The logical, mindful part of my brain had gone offline. I was consumed by a want that felt like need, and nothing else mattered.

I got high for the last time just a month later. What changed? What made me teachable?

## Step Zero

Hitting bottom is a moment of reckoning, sometimes called a moment of clarity. It is when our denial dissolves in the backwash of our actions. On January 5, 1986, the consequences of my addiction became impossible to ignore. It wasn't the first time I'd seen that drugs were causing me problems. I had sold my treasured instruments, trading music for drugs. I was living in my car with everything I owned: a bag of dirty clothes, a dull syringe, and a pistol. Any of these might have been a bottom for someone else, but that morning I was still clinging to the illusion of power and control.

An addict chases immediate relief and pushes away thoughts of the consequences, convinced the benefit outweighs the cost—until the pain becomes too great to bear. My brother Richard was also an addict. When he gave me my first taste of opiates, he offered a bit of advice: "Pete, you'll probably throw up, but don't worry, it's just part of the high." I took it as a life lesson.

A bottom is a moment of surrender, when the pain we are in exceeds the pain we are trying to avoid. For some, waking up sick is enough. For others, it takes the loss of a job or relationship, incarceration, hospitalization, or homelessness. Tragically, for Richard and others, the bottom is death. I was incarcerated when his pain became too much to bear, and suicide seemed to be the only surrender he could find. My family had cut off contact a year earlier, and I didn't hear about his death until I got out.

On the morning of January 5, 1986, I sat in my car, feeling sick and defeated. Too weak to continue, I looked at my gun and thought about where I could get the money to "get well" again. There had been times when I had romanticized the addict life, even taking pride in the crimes I'd committed. Those days were gone. My last robbery had been sticking up a man selling bags of oranges on a freeway off-ramp. I sped away like I'd robbed a bank, trying to outrun my shame. Now, even shoplifting seemed scary.

I sat in a quagmire of dope sickness and despair, the gun heavy in my hand. I didn't know how to stop using, and I couldn't imagine a life without drugs. I thought of Richard. Just a month earlier, he had sat in his car before ending his life with a bullet.

Looking down the barrel, I saw only loneliness and despair.

Something shifted. A will to live broke through the cloud of self-centered fear. I didn't want to die. I didn't even want the temporary relief of the next fix. All I wanted was a place to lie down and kick my habit in peace. In that moment, I saw it clearly: drugs were the reason I was in that car, in that state. The fleeting comfort they offered was inevitably followed by deeper suffering. That small hope of peace became a turning point.

I worried about forgetting this truth. Addiction is called a disease of forgetfulness, where euphoric recall eclipses the pain. I was afraid this sudden clarity would fade. It had before. I would not survive another cycle.

How could I keep this realization alive?

For the first time, fear, loneliness, and despair were not problems to escape, but experiences of value. I wanted to imprint this moment in my body—to let it become a resource and a lasting catalyst. Without realizing it, I was nurturing mindfulness, fully present with my suffering and guided by good intention.

I took care to remember the taste of that loneliness: my aching bones and squirming intestines, the cold fear in every pore. The visceral memory became a treasured counterpoint to the fantasies of getting high that inevitably return.

My mind had long been a refuge, freeing me from the confines of my body and helping me bypass the emotions that overwhelmed me. But in the car that morning, something different happened. I turned toward the feelings rather than away from them. I sank deeper into my body, fully present for the raw sensations of the moment, burrowing beneath my stories and thoughts of escape. My mind and body no longer felt divided. For a moment, I experienced an embodied mind and a mindful body.

I later learned that the Buddha called this "mindfulness of body." His phrase, "mindfulness of the body in the body," points less to thinking about the body and more to inhabiting it.* Insight isn't a concept. It's the embodied experience when "oh shit" becomes "aha."

I had allowed thoughts of getting high to drive my actions. First I entertained them; then they became an obsession. The clarity of that moment in the Pinto gave me a new tool. When the thought of getting high arose, I listened to my body and remembered how it felt in that car. The physical memory became an antidote to euphoric recall.

---

* Mindfulness of the body is the First Establishment of Mindfulness in the Satipaṭṭhāna Sutta, which offers specific practices and a more nuanced exploration of this way of being. See Thich Nhat Hanh, *Transformation and Healing: Discourse of the Four Establishments of Mindfulness* (Parallax Press, 2002).

Instead of fixating on an imagined rush or release, analyzing the craving, or negotiating with it, I learned to associate the thought of getting high with its inevitable result: the full-body despair and fear I had felt so deeply that morning. Turning from mind to body grounded me and proved liberating. I was no longer a victim of the obsession.

Every time I relapsed, my body had tried to warn me: a tightening in the gut, a hollow feeling, a closing throat, a weight in the chest. I drowned those sensations in a stream of thoughts to bypass them. The addict mind is skilled at denial and rationalization. The gut check has become invaluable for me.

When I stopped resisting and embraced painful moments, fear, shame, and pain became noble, revealing both the cause of suffering and the possibility of its end. Over time, the imagined relief of using became linked to the embodied memory of that January morning, what I now think of as my "Pinto moment." This capacity to rewire our thoughts, responses, and behavior is now understood as neuroplasticity.

My insight didn't come from a book—no one could teach me how to surrender. It arose from a moment of presence, stripped of excuses and delusion. When I was beaten down enough to surrender my belief in drugs as a solution, a medicine, or a superpower, it became unmistakably clear that they were a cause of suffering.

I think of this as "step zero," the threshold many of us cross before recovery can truly begin. It is the clarity born of surrender that informs a commitment to abstinence.

Not using became freedom from the suffering I was living in. No matter how difficult things might become, I knew drugs would only make them worse. Abstinence was no longer a loss or a sacrifice. It became a source of joy.

How strange. The intoxicants I had mistaken for happiness were revealed as the source of my suffering, while abstinence, once feared as suffering, became the source of true happiness.

## Appropriate Attention

Profound moments of insight often fade as we are swept along in the stream of life. How do we keep them alive? The program has a clear answer for this question.

Surrender is a funny word, usually associated with defeat. But in Zen and recovery, it is letting go, not giving up. It is a beautiful form of empowerment: acting from choice rather than reactive conditioning. With awareness, we learn to let go of resistance rather than feeding or fighting it. We loosen the grip of rigid views, of our ideas about how things are supposed to be when we are at odds with the way they are. Surrender is a shift in perception, a softening that allows a new perspective to appear.

Hitting bottom gave me the willingness to do whatever it took to stay clean. I never wanted to feel that way again. If there was an answer in the rooms of recovery, I wanted to be there. I had nowhere else to turn. The desperation that once drove my addiction became "the gift of desperation," nourishing my commitment to stay clean "no matter what." I understood clearly that no matter how bad things got, drugs would ultimately make things worse.

With the surrender, I became teachable. I returned to Twelve-Step meetings, hungry for guidance rather than intoxicants. I was ready to learn, and it no longer mattered how you dressed, where you had been, what drugs you used, or if you had tattoos. If you knew something that could help me stay clean, I wanted to hear it. Anyone and everyone was my teacher.

Staying clean became my number one priority. I was encouraged to use the program the way I'd used drugs, and I knew what that meant. I was told to go to ninety meetings in ninety days, call another addict daily, get a sponsor, and read the literature daily. I wondered if I was trading one crutch for another. It felt cultish to live my life around the program rather than fitting the program into my life. But I was actually being trained in what the Buddha called appropriate attention. Keeping the program first was like following the breath in meditation. I learned to notice what is deepening and encouraging recovery and what pulls me away. I was replacing chemical dependency with a path of freedom.

In the Buddha's time, buildings were held together with wooden pegs. Over years of rain and weather, these pegs would rot. If you pulled out a rotten peg without replacing it, the whole structure could collapse. But if you tapped in a new peg, it naturally pushed the old one out. Addiction and recovery were like that for me. Removing drugs left a vacuum that pulled me back into the vortex of old habit energy. Recovery gave me a new peg. I replaced old ways of thinking and living with new ones and committed myself as if my life depended on it—because it did. Like an addict looking for a fix, I focused on what I could use.

Happiness comes and goes. With mind training, otherwise known as appropriate attention, we can learn to refresh and renew it. Conditions for happiness are always available if we look deeply. My experience with Zen has shown that it is always possible to generate a feeling of happiness. That's a tall order when someone dies or when depression takes hold. Yet I heard the same wisdom in early recovery: Any day clean is a good day. Happiness is relative. Things could always be worse.

Most of the time, happiness feels conditional: "I'll be happy when...," or "I'm happy because...." Yet even with grief, illness, or injustice, we have the capacity to recognize and water seeds of joy. Happiness isn't entirely dependent on outer circumstances. As my teacher Thay said,* "Sometimes your smile is the result of your happiness. Sometimes your happiness is the result of your smile." Sometimes feelings of well-being are as simple as experiencing abstinence or breathing freely.

---

* Thich Nhat Hanh (1926–2022) was known by his students as *Thay*, meaning "teacher."

The greatest obstacle to contentment is dwelling on what seems wrong. My untrained mind is brilliantly critical. It is gifted at spotting what's missing and consumed by whatever feels off.

We are apparently wired with this negativity bias. The nervous system constantly scans for threats, and our mind interprets these inputs at lightning speed. When our system is activated, we shift into survival mode—pure reactivity. This ancient survival mechanism once ensured our survival. Nowadays, it often works against us, keeping us in a world of fear and lack rather than abundance. Neuroscience shows that negative experiences generate more brain activity than positive or neutral ones. That explains how a single hurt seems to eclipse everything good in our lives.

Appropriate attention is an antidote. It is mindful awareness guided by Right Intention: our capacity for healing, harmony, and freedom. It reminds us that we'd rather be happy than angry. The ground of happiness is always available in the here and now.

Being present with focus and care allows me to be both an observer and a participant. I notice thoughts and feelings with curiosity and recognize the stories I tell myself about the way things are. I begin to see whether I am reacting or responding; whether I'm moving toward connection or slipping into the old patterns of separation.

Reactions arise in a heartbeat but easily spiral into a self-perpetuating loop. A single moment becomes the whole story. We turn a snapshot into a movie and replay it endlessly. Each time, amplifying our distress until it becomes a spiral of suffering that feels inescapable. With mindfulness and appropriate attention, we recover the capacity to respond. Our grip loosens. Spaciousness returns. Surrender, reframing, and reorienting—choice—become possible again.

The Twelve Steps, like mindfulness meditation, train awareness and discernment. They help soften our negativity bias and transform afflicted states into something beneficial. Simply noticing reactivity opens the space for a response. We train responsiveness rather than reflex. Freedom is not found in controlling triggers. It is in recognizing and showing up for our afflicted states. That's where healing and growth happen.

## Walking the Path

The Four Noble Truths and the Twelve Steps are both paths to spiritual awakening that invite us to turn toward suffering rather than away from it. That may seem counterintuitive, but it is practical and immensely rewarding. Each offers a path through the wilderness of life and a way to make good use of suffering.

This is where the path becomes concrete.

> **Step One:** *We admitted that we are powerless over our addiction (affliction) and that our lives had become unmanageable.*

The First Step names what I had been fighting for years: powerlessness. My life had clearly become unmanageable. But what did powerless mean?

I had never considered powerlessness before. I had to learn to recognize it. When I became mindful of my body, I noticed the clues: muscles tightening, breath accelerating, blood pressure rising as I became angry, impatient, intolerant, or frustrated. Once aware, I could trace these reactions back to a feeling of powerlessness—usually because reality didn't match my wants or expectations. Seeing that, the antidote was acceptance. This is just the way it is right now—a fleeting moment in the stream of my life. If I am clean, healthy, and alive, it is still a good day.

What we resist persists and grows stronger. Have you ever tried to hold a beach ball underwater? With the First Step, I discovered a new way of engaging with life. Instead of fighting, I learned to stop and release. Where I once said "fuck it" and checked out with drugs, I learned to say "no big deal" and let go.

Admitting I am powerless over my addiction meant accepting that I cannot drink or use, even socially. For an addict, one always leads to more. Powerlessness is not an abstract concept; it is always over something specific. Recognizing my powerlessness over addiction led me to a deeper question: What do I actually have power over? I began to question my long-held assumption that I had power over people, places, and things.

The Buddha looked deeply and discovered something very different: nothing exists as a separate, independent entity. Everything is a conglomeration of conditions. We are not just ourselves; we contain the DNA of our parents and ancestors. Our bodies are composed of billions of cells, each made of countless atoms. We include not only human cells but also nonhuman cells, the microorganisms that help digest our food. We contain water, minerals, air, and energy. Even our thoughts and perceptions are shaped by teachers, culture, history, trauma, ideology, and inheritance.

Nothing arises on its own. Everything manifests only when conditions come together. The Buddha called this "dependent origination." We tend to think in simple cause-and-effect terms, but that too is a habit of dualistic thinking. One cause is never enough to bring about an effect. Every cause is also an effect, and every effect becomes a cause of something else—the chain is endless. Sounds like powerlessness, doesn't it?

Normal perception defies this awareness. Of course, we "think" there is a single cause for a result. "I" type this word, and it manifests on the page! But what appears to be a simple, single action is made up of innumerable causes and conditions. This page exists because of trees, ink, electricity, generations of invention, and countless people I'll never meet. Even the act of typing a sentence depends on a web of conditions: a body, a mind, electricity, tools, teachers, and countless people and places that made this moment possible.

We can influence our actions, but most conditions shaping our lives lie far beyond our control and reach back generations. This is not fatalism; it's freedom. When we release the illusion of control, we are free to meet life as it is, with humility, compassion, and awe. I don't have to manage the world anymore. What a relief! The First Step helped me apply the principle of surrender I had touched in Step Zero to the rest of my life.

We interpret our lives through the stories we make up about them. Before long, we mistake those views for reality. Our minds label an event "unacceptable," and we suffer, convinced that it is. Thankfully, our stories can be edited. We don't have to like the way things are or approve of them to accept them. What we call surrender is actually a shift in perception.

Our deepest addiction may be to our own thoughts—endlessly ruminating, comparing, judging, replaying what happened or what never did. We begin to see ourselves as victims of fate, the world, genetics, or upbringing, shaped by forces beyond our control. In this way, we can become attached to suffering itself, holding onto pain as if it were a prized possession. Resentment is a perfect example. We replay the tapes, rehearse what we could or should have said, and share our outrage as if justification might bring relief. Instead, we reinforce our attachment to the very pain we're complaining about.

Harmony heals. Resistance is dis-ease. With awareness and acceptance, we can reorient toward well-being rather than ill-being. This is the practice of Right View, Right Effort, and Right Mindfulness described in the Fourth Noble Truth.

The world isn't out to get me. I have a program, a practice, tools of recovery, and support. I don't have to fight what I don't like. Powerlessness can lead me to gratitude rather than unmanageability. With mindfulness, I can soften reactivity. Agitation becomes an invitation to harmonize. Stopping and releasing, the practice of surrender, has become central to both my recovery and meditation practice.

Both the Buddha and the program remind us that we can change our view. We can choose freedom over fixation. Surrender can feel like a superpower. With Right Mindfulness, freedom is always available. Transforming suffering is spiritual alchemy.

## Coming to Our Senses

Sometimes, all it takes is a breeze on my skin to remind me I'm alive. Not because it's dramatic but because it's not. It's just there, and I'm here to feel it. My friend Cathy used to say that a gentle breeze felt like surrender. Every physical sensation carries a feeling tone: pleasant, unpleasant, or neutral. The Buddha taught this in the Second Establishment of Mindfulness, mindfulness of feeling.

Our senses receive a constant stream of information, and the nervous system rapidly filters it, assessing safety or danger before we are consciously aware of it. We respond viscerally. A warm smile feels safe, and the body relaxes. It is experienced as a pleasant feeling. If the nervous system perceives a threat, even a garden hose mistakenly identified as a snake, the body shifts into survival mode and an unpleasant fear arises. Much of our experience falls somewhere in between, what the Buddha described as neutral feeling.

As I write this, I pause to practice. I notice the sensation of air on my skin. My mind quickly labels it air and dismisses it. Staying with the sensation, it first feels neutral—neither too hot nor too cold. As I feel the air move, I notice a subtle coolness that I recognize as pleasant. When I first practiced this teaching, neutral feelings were the hardest to notice because they are so easily overlooked. One of the gifts of mindfulness is that neutral feelings, when noticed, often reveal quiet forms of pleasure. My cotton T-shirt is neither too tight nor too loose. It's soft, and for most of the day, I'm unaware of its contact with my skin. With attention, the absence of discomfort becomes the pleasant sensation of soft cotton resting on my body.

Practicing in this way, we begin to see that feelings arise and pass. A neutral feeling fades as a pleasant one emerges. Like all things, they are impermanent. With training, we learn to appreciate and sustain pleasant feelings without clinging to them. We also learn to recognize and care for unpleasant feelings sooner, helping them soften into a neutral state.

This simple shift of attention is what the Buddha described as Right Effort on the Noble Eightfold Path. Right Effort, also called Right Diligence, is the energy we use to cultivate what leads to well-being and to care for and transform the causes of suffering. It is not striving or forcing, but the steady, compassionate energy of mindfulness. Traditionally, Right Effort consists of four practices:

1. Preventing unwholesome states from arising
2. Transforming unwholesome states that have arisen
3. Cultivating wholesome states that have not yet arisen
4. Nourishing and maintaining the wholesome states that have presently arisen

The Second Step in recovery echoes this path with its own invitation to healing:

> **Step Two:** *We came to believe that a power greater than ourselves could restore us to sanity.*

Coming to believe in a greater power is a big deal. For the first time, I found comfort without intoxicants. I came to believe in life after drugs. This wasn't blind faith; I had evidence that the program was working for me. Though I struggled with the Judeo-Christian language of recovery and the idea of a higher power, I came to see the program itself as a power greater than myself. The group was greater than the sum of its parts: direction, wisdom, and support emerged from our collective. Together, we were doing what none of us could do alone.

Using the program as a higher power was practical and served me well for a time. It wasn't the be-all and end-all, but it was undeniably a positive force in my life. Over time, other understandings of a higher power emerged, including love and nature. Eventually, through meditation, I began to experience mindfulness, a caring quality of attention that is always available, as a power greater than myself.

In my experience, mindfulness embodies loving kindness, compassion, and curiosity. It is a connective energy that helps me come home to spacious well-being, where I can respond rather than react. In this way, mindfulness is greater than my small, egoic self.

Sanity is often defined as "thinking and behaving in a normal and rational manner." Is that as good as it gets? In early recovery, the Second Step reminded me that I had a path and support. It was no longer me versus the world; there was an us. Sanity meant using the tools and resources that were available.

Restoration begins with clarity. People come to recovery hurting and in need of help, but many stop taking the medicine once they experience some relief. These days, I think of sanity as the restoration of clarity and willingness. Clarity is the antidote to unwillingness—and willingness is what keeps the medicine working.

Trying to think my way into recovery had never worked. I'd quit many times, only to talk myself into picking up again. As Richard Rohr said, "We do not think ourselves into new ways of living; we live ourselves into new ways of thinking." This time, I surrendered my resistance and took the suggested actions. In letting go, I found the freedom I had been chasing all along.

I was beginning to hear the music of healing instead of getting snagged by the words. When the lyrics didn't make sense, the melody carried me. I used to think that drinking was my father's problem, and I was somehow hipper for being a drug addict. But when my life hung in the balance, those labels lost their meaning. Addict or alcoholic became as irrelevant as my struggles with the word "God." In practical terms, any mind-altering substance would derail my life. The simple clarity of "Don't get loaded no matter what" became a guiding light. Drink the medicine, not the poison.

The Second Step was an antidote to my obsession to use, but other urges quickly appeared. I kept chasing happiness. I thought it was something outside of me. We're conditioned to believe happiness lies in the future. Advertising reinforces the idea that we'll be okay once we get something we don't yet have. Believing that I need something external to feel okay inside is a form of delusion—or insanity in the parlance of Twelve-Step recovery. Even when I get what I want, the satisfaction is temporary. If it disappoints me, I want something else; if it fulfills me, I fear losing it.

There's an old saying: happiness isn't getting what you want; it's wanting what you have.* What if we already had enough and nothing essential was lacking? With a restoration of clarity, we can live from abundance rather than scarcity, with appreciation for what's already here. All too often, I didn't recognize the value of something—or someone—until it was gone.

For me, peace and happiness arise from within, and surrender is the key. With attention and intention, we can care for our toxic states of mind, and that itself is a kind of happiness.

Restoration means returning something to its original condition. What is our original condition? For much of my life, I believed there was something fundamentally wrong or broken in me. Our culture urges us to strive, achieve, and prove ourselves, promising happiness as the payoff for effort. But what if we are already worthy? What if well-being is not something to earn but our birthright?

## Our Original Nature

I came to meditation like I came to drugs—looking for a fix. I wanted peace and craved enlightenment. In time, the practice revealed that what I was seeking wasn't outside of me. It was my original nature, already here. I began to see the difference between setting a clear intention and chasing an expectation. An intention

---

* Hyman Judah Schachtel, *The Real Enjoyment of Living* (Dutton, 1954), 37.

is aligned with our values; an expectation clings to a particular outcome. Intention and aspiration feel spacious; expectation and craving often feel tight.

Mindfulness is a remembering—a return to our original nature. We don't sit to find peace; peace is already here. We are already enough. There is nothing to seek.

Even now, you might pause. Just for a moment. Notice what's here: The breath. The body. The quiet conditions of peace are already present. You are likely clothed, sheltered, fed, and safe. These are already conditions for peace and happiness. If peace is available in this moment, you know another moment of peace is possible.

Mindfulness and the Second Step are coming home to a well-being that doesn't depend on external conditions. The Buddha observed that the mind is always searching outside itself and never feels fulfilled. That sounds a lot like addiction. The searching mind is part of being human; mindfulness meditation is a shift from thought to awareness. In practice, this is a deep surrender. When the searching pauses, I come home to the present moment and rediscover the ground of being—spacious, steady, and at ease.

This resonates with my understanding of the Second Step. Mindfulness is always available; it is the essence of restoration. It meets suffering with gentle presence; like a hand cradling an injured finger it heals with kindness.

With mindfulness of the body and feelings, my attention becomes more refined. I can often recognize afflicted states as they arise, before they sweep me away. Caring for these states, there is nothing to fix. The steady presence of mindfulness soothes emotions and quiets the divisive mind that clings to a separate self and amplifies suffering.

It's counterintuitive, but the parts of us that are hurt and fearful are the ones most in need of love. My initial response to pain or perceived threat is often fear, which quickly turns into anger. Stub a toe and watch what happens. Cursing and harsh self-talk add insult to injury. There's a teaching that says when your house is on fire, it's better to put out the fire than to chase after whoever lit it. A gentle touch brings more relief than blame.

Knowing how unkind I can be, even to myself, it was a revelation to discover that my true nature, my original nature, is love. This ran counter to a lifetime of stories I'd been telling myself. We don't have to become loving; we return to love by recognizing and letting go of what isn't.

After Siddhartha Gautama's awakening under the bodhi tree, people began calling him the Buddha, meaning the awakened one. They could see it in his face, posture, and presence. The Buddha wondered whether awakening could be shared. He concluded that all beings possess this capacity. We call it Buddha nature—the capacity to awaken.

This can sound like something to attain, but Buddha nature is already within us. It is our original goodness, our teachability, our capacity to learn and to help one another. It's one addict listening to another with compassion and care. It is the part of us that reaches out in pain, to soothe rather than punish. Awakened nature is recovery nature; it is the capacity for freedom from active addiction.

The insanity addressed in the Second Step is the belief that things should be different from the way they are. This includes inner states as well as people, places, and things. It's a view rooted in self-obsession: what I want and how I think life ought to be. Accepting life as it is in this moment doesn't make me a victim or a slave to circumstances. My freedom lies in how I engage and respond.

"I have arrived, I am home" is one of four Dharma seals that form the foundation of the Plum Village Tradition of Engaged Buddhism.* Stopping, releasing, and arriving is the heart of our

---

* The other three are "Go as a river," "The times and truths inter-are," and "Ripening, moment by moment."

practice. Home is here and now, wherever we are. When we stop running and arrive, the miracle and mystery of life are available.

Let's make this real. You don't have to take it on faith. Pause and see what's here. Become aware of your body—sitting, standing, walking, or lying down. You are in contact with the earth and the sky. Your lungs breathe. Your heart beats, sustaining your life. Without effort, your body digests, nourishes, and releases. Your eyes see; your ears hear. Your mind receives, interprets, and makes meaning.

This astonishing constellation we call "me" is awake, aware.

Here and now, we are nourishing recovery and our awakening. There is wonder; there is mystery; there is awe.

You might pause and let Thay's words accompany a few breaths:

*I have arrived, I am home.*
*In the here and in the now.*
*I am solid, I am free*
*in the ultimate I dwell.*

Stopping and arriving takes practice, but it can be done gently, with joy and ease.

What is this?

## The Two Truths

In recovery, we're encouraged to be "a part of" rather than "apart from." Is that a choice, or something like grace, unexpected and unearned? We may experience moments of profound connection in meditation or in nature, when the boundary between self and other dissolves. It can feel like oneness and deep belonging. Yet even the word "oneness" is conceptual—it implies twoness and separation. Nirvana is not something we can capture in words; it is the direct experience of reality, free from labels and notions. The Buddha called this "suchness."

Our experience of reality is shaped by perception. Like the parable of the blind men and the elephant, each touching a different part and drawing different conclusions, what we perceive depends on where we stand and what we touch.

Buddhist teachings speak of two truths, complementary ways of seeing that help us relate more wisely to life. Conventional truth is relative and conditional—the truth of everyday experience. I am me and you are you. There is a past, present, and future. Things appear to arise and pass away. Thay called this the historical dimension, where we function through names, roles, and pairs of opposites. The second is ultimate truth, what Thay called the ultimate dimension. It is nondual and unconditioned. The one contains the many, and the many contain the one.

Time is a useful convention. Labels are necessary. Words like good and bad, up and down, right and wrong help us navigate conventional reality. In the ultimate, boundaries soften. What appears separate is revealed as interwoven. The ultimate is not better than the historical, nor separate from it. They interpenetrate like waves and water, only distinct in the way we look.

Looking deeply, we see they are not two. Dwelling only in the absolute is not ultimate awakening. The two truths dance together. If we lose touch with the historical dimension, we are likely to end up in prison or a mental hospital. Knowing we are all one doesn't mean I can sleep in your bed or take your money. Touching the absolute reshapes my understanding of the relative and how I live. More often, we mistake the conventional for the ultimate—believing our labels tell the whole truth.

When we dislike someone, it can be hard to see anything good in them. A single hurt can eclipse years of friendship. A bad moment can color an entire day. Our conditioned mind treats emotions as absolutes, as if sadness negates joy or joy erases sorrow.

With mindfulness, we begin to see how opposites depend on one another. Sound and silence arise together. Sadness and gladness are two sides of the same coin. This is a glimpse of the ultimate dimension. Even "up" depends on perspective. What is up in North America is not up in India. In space, there is no up or down; the question disappears entirely.

Right View, sometimes called Right Understanding, is seeing things as they are: not fixed or separate, but as living, changing processes. A Zen teaching attributed to Qingyuan Weixin describes this shift: first there is a mountain, then there is no mountain, and then there is a mountain again. At first, the mountain is simply a mountain—our idea of it. Then there is no mountain: we see through the concept and recognize it as soil, minerals, plants, water, and time. Finally, there is a mountain again, but now we know it is made of non-mountain elements. We can use the word mountain without being trapped by it.

The two truths help us dwell in both realms. In the relative dimension, I am Pete. I have a birthday, responsibilities, and a story. But in the ultimate dimension, Pete is made of non-Pete elements—earth, water, air, and energy. Cells arise and pass away every moment. My ancestors live in my body; their choices, traumas, hopes, and resilience flow through me. Even my capacity to heal and recover depends on countless conditions: my sponsor, my sangha, my teachers, the food I eat, the air I breathe.

Emotions arise in the historical dimension, yet they insist they are the ultimate truth. In conventional perception, I may feel lonely, but in the absolute, I am never alone. I am connected to all beings across space and time, inseparable from everything.

We can read about Right View, listen to Dharma talks, and watch videos, but without engaged practice, it all remains theoretical. Our thoughts are seductive, and our dependency on them runs very deep. We need direct experience to develop an understanding that is more than notional. It can be hard to distinguish a view from reality when we mistake our thoughts for the way things actually are.

The two truths are a skillful means to explore the complex nature of reality—not a final answer.

## Three Treasures

When I was new in recovery, desperation opened my mind and helped me overcome objections that had previously derailed me. The word "God" was one of them. Turning my will and my life over to something was another. Another surrender opened the way.

> **Step Three:** *We made a decision to turn our will and our lives over to the care of God, as we understood him.*

The first three steps lay a foundation that supports the deeper work that follows. When I was new, this is how I understood them: the First Step taught me to turn toward the program when difficulty arose. The Second Step helped me trust the program as a viable path. The Third Step was a commitment to live that path—something far deeper than abstinence alone.

The word "God" was still charged for me. This step gave me the creeps. I had to loosen my views to find a way through, so I substituted "the program." It had proven to be a path to freedom, and I made it my top priority. With Right Mindfulness and Right Intention, I committed to Right Action. At the time, I called this program action, aligning my thoughts and behavior with what nourishes recovery and letting go of what does not.

By now, you may have noticed how the Noble Truths support one another. Right Intention informs Right Action, which is how intention takes form in the world. With Right View, we see that everything is composite and interdependent. The Steps work this way, too. The surrender of Step One creates the conditions for all that follows. From the clarity of Step Two arises the decision of Step Three. Each step, in its own way, deepens the surrender.

Over time, Step Three became a commitment to intentional living, which is central to the Eightfold Path. Commitment feels scary when I fear failure, but this isn't about perfection. There will always be detours. Like a GPS, we recalibrate, guided by a north star. I don't walk the path to be "good" or earn heaven; I walk it because it feels right.

I am committed to using every aspect of my life to support recovery and awakening. In everyday situations, I pause to consider, "What is the next program action here?" Over time, I came to associate the spirit of the program and my understanding of a higher power with love. I often pause to ask, "What does love look like in this situation?" It's a kind of koan practice, with no fixed answer.

Working the Third Step had practical consequences. At first, I stopped shoplifting, something I had once considered a skill. When I found work, it was a telephone sales hustle, selling overpriced copier toner to businesses by promising prizes that never materialized. I made good money, but it felt no different from hustling stolen goods in active addiction. Though I was clean, the deception didn't align with my new values. That realization led me to find more ethical work.

This is what Buddhists call Right Livelihood—earning a living in ways that cause no harm. I took a job in a warehouse, eventually moving into electronics sales. Military clients were among the largest customers, but as an old peacenik, I declined accounts related to weaponry. This, too, felt like Right Livelihood. I didn't need a rulebook. I was reconnecting with my core values.

As the Dharma began informing my recovery, I started to see the Steps through a Buddhist lens. The powerlessness and unmanageability of the First Step reflected forgetfulness: being swept up in reactivity and self-pity. The restoration to sanity in the Second Step was a return to the restorative energy of mindfulness. The Third Step became a vow to live in mindfulness.

And the God thing? Buddhist faith isn't based on belief in the unseen. The Buddha encouraged people to test his teachings in their own lives. Twelve-Step recovery works the same way: the results show up in how we live. The Dharma and the Steps aren't theoretical; they're experiential and evidence based.

The tools of recovery include meetings, sponsorship, literature, service, and working the Steps. The tools of the Dharma include ethical living, mindful breathing, meditation, sangha, and weaving awareness into daily life. Together, they form a complete path.

The Judeo-Christian language of the Steps still gives me pause. It took me years to notice how deeply patriarchal language had been normalized in my own thinking. I'm grateful that many fellowships are revising language to be more inclusive. We are encouraged to find a higher power of our own understanding. Following Thay's example, I will vary the pronouns I use when referring to God. I mean no offense and invite you to substitute whatever language fits for you.

## Taking Refuge

The sudden death of my seventeen-year-old stepson, David, in 2002 led me to Deer Park Monastery and the practice of mindfulness. Grief has become an endless river flowing through my life of recovery and practice. At times it becomes raging rapids, or a whirlpool pulling me into seemingly bottomless depths. At other times, it flows as a river of awakening, carrying me toward a deeper sense of meaning and purpose.

I met David's mother, Jackie, when I was five years into recovery, and we married the following year. David was five when I met him; his sister, Vanessa, was seven. I learned a great deal about love while parenting David and Vanessa. I remember sitting on the couch in the early days, both children on my lap, feeling an indescribable connection—pure, innocent, ancient, and protective. Vanessa later moved in with her father during high school, while David made a life with us in San Diego. David and I formed a deep bond. He was a musician who gigged with his band, the captain of the wrestling team, a surfer, a gamer, funny, and full of life.

When David died suddenly from an undiagnosed heart condition, my world was turned upside down and inside out. This, the most devastating event of my life, became a profound teacher. Without his death, this book would never have come to be.

The shocking finality of his death rattled my bones and woke me to the fragility and impermanence of life. Everything I once considered important evaporated in an instant. Alongside the pain came a regret—not that I hadn't loved him but that I hadn't been more present. I had been busy parenting: reminding him to make his bed, brush his teeth, do his homework, finish his chores. I was preparing him for a future that would never arrive. I longed for more moments of simply being together, as two souls on a shared journey, appreciating the miracle of life and our connection.

Over time, I learned to care for grief. That doesn't mean it stopped hurting; I learned to "compost" the suffering and find value within it. With wise care, even the unfathomable loss of a child can become noble suffering: the kind of suffering that wakes us up.

After David's death, Jackie dug deep. One of the books she read was *No Death, No Fear* by Thich Nhat Hanh.* I was reluctant when she suggested visiting a nearby monastery in Thay's Plum Village Zen tradition. Twelve-Step recovery had been my entire world for sixteen years, and I was afraid to step outside that familiar container. Still, I agreed to go, mainly to support her. My life changed in ways I could not have imagined.

Though my initial visit to the monastery wasn't love at first sight, a casual conversation with a kind monk and the discovery of *Be Free Where You Are* in the gift shop drew me back.† I had explored Buddhism before, but it felt abstract until I read *Be Free Where You Are.* Thay's teachings were clear, practical, and immediately resonant with my experience of recovery. I had been taught

---

* Thich Nhat Hanh, *No Death, No Fear: Comforting Wisdom for Life* (Riverhead Books, 2003).

† Thich Nhat Hanh, *Be Free Where You Are* (Parallax Press, 2002).

to apply the program to all my affairs; Thay was offering the Dharma in the same spirit.

As I practiced mindfulness, I learned how to show up for life with greater presence. Offering my whole being to each moment feels like the most authentic way I can honor David and live my love for him. With mindfulness, this love doesn't stagnate when I can't communicate it to him directly—it grows and finds new ways to flow. I think of it as music that can be made from all the sounds, including silence.

Inspired, I wanted to go deeper into the teachings and practice of mindfulness. I was all in and wanted to declare myself a Buddhist. I imagined how satisfying it would be to write "Buddhist" on a form that asked for my religion or announce it to friends. At the time, I didn't understand that Buddhism is a practice, not a belief system or identity to adopt. Thay encouraged us to honor our root traditions and use mindfulness practice to deepen that, but I wasn't interested in my Jewish roots then.

When I asked how to become a Buddhist, I was told, "You're a Buddhist when you say you are." I laughed. People in Twelve-Step recovery said the same thing about being an addict or alcoholic. Unsatisfied, I searched online and learned that traditionally, becoming a Buddhist involves taking refuge in the Three Jewels. I immediately recited the words: "I take refuge in the Buddha. I take refuge in the Dharma. I take refuge in the Sangha." They were only words. It felt like a hollow formality.

Then I encountered Thay's chant, "The Three Refuges," and taking refuge became a lived experience. This chant became a guide for my life and recovery.

### The Three Refuges Chant

*I take refuge in the Buddha,*
*the one who shows me the way in this life.*
*I take refuge in the Dharma,*

*the way of understanding and of love.*
*I take refuge in the Sangha,*
*the community that lives in harmony and awareness.*

*Dwelling in the refuge of Buddha,*
*I clearly see the path of light and beauty in the world.*
*Dwelling in the refuge of Dharma,*
*I learn to open many doors on the path of transformation.*
*Dwelling in the refuge of Sangha,*
*shining light that supports me, keeping my practice free of obstruction.*

*Taking refuge in the Buddha in myself,*
*I aspire to help all people recognize their own awakened nature,*
*realizing the mind of love.*
*Taking refuge in the Dharma in myself,*
*I aspire to help all people fully master the ways of practice*
*and walk together on the path of liberation.*
*Taking refuge in the Sangha in myself,*
*I aspire to help all people build fourfold communities,*
*to embrace all beings and support their transformation.**

For me, the Buddha, Dharma, and Sangha parallel the program, the Steps, and the fellowship. Taking refuge felt akin to the Third Step, and more agreeable than turning my will and life over to a God I didn't understand. I came to see awakened nature as the energy of love, our inherent wisdom and teachability. This awakened nature is also our recovery nature: the capacity to transform old habits, compost suffering, and help others. The Buddha, the one who shows the way, became the program. The Dharma, the teachings and tools of transformation, were the Steps. And the Sangha was the fellowship.

* Thich Nhat Hanh, *Chanting from the Heart*, vol. 1, (Parallax Press, 2023), 108.

When I first came to the program, I felt like an outsider. There was "me" and "them," and I wasn't sure I belonged. At some point, "they" became "us." I was part of the fellowship—giving and receiving, connected to people around the world committed to helping one another. As I worked the Steps and sponsored others, the program became alive in me. I was helping protect and sustain it. The Three Refuges unfolded in the same way. In the Sangha, we are more than the sum of our parts. Vulnerability becomes strength, and collective wisdom emerges.

As we live the program and practice mindfulness, we begin to care for others and want all beings to find freedom from addiction and suffering. This is called *bodhicitta*, the mind of awakening. Dwelling in the refuges, we receive support and naturally offer it in return.

Mindfulness, the quality of caring attention available to all of us, supports this entire process. With appropriate attention and intention, it nourishes every aspect of the Noble Eightfold Path and all the factors of awakening, naturally giving rise to openness and curiosity. This brings us to the second factor of awakening: investigation.

# THE SECOND FACTOR OF AWAKENING:

# Investigation

## Opening the Buddha Eye

This factor points to an active, curious inquiry into our experience. We explore the causes, conditions, and patterns revealed by mindfulness. The Sanskrit term for this quality is *dharmavichaya* (Pāli: *dhammavicaya*), often translated as "investigation of dharmas."

*Dharma* with a capital "D" refers to the Buddha's teachings. With a small "d," *dharmas* are the moment-to-moment elements of experience—thoughts, feelings, bodily sensations, and mental states. Investigation is the practice of meeting these phenomena with interest and care, allowing the fruit of understanding to grow. Mindfulness meditation is a stabilizing practice that clarifies the mind, creating conditions for wholesome investigation.

Thay described meditation as a bird with two wings: stopping (*shamatha*) and looking deeply (*vipassana*). Both are needed for flight, or in this case, the fruit of insight. We begin by stopping and calming, but thoughts, feelings, and memories inevitably arise during meditation. When settled in calm abiding, we hold them in spacious awareness, allowing insight to arise. We look deeply into their nature with the gentle energy of investigation.

Sometimes investigation unfolds most vividly through direct experience. In 2008, I traveled to India for a retreat with Thich Nhat Hanh called "In the Footsteps of the Buddha." It was a wonderful experience, lovingly organized by Shantum Seth, an Indian

Dharma teacher in the Plum Village tradition. After watching the sun rise on the Ganges River, we made our way to Sarnath, the historic site where the Buddha gave his first teaching after enlightenment. There, on the quiet grounds where the Dharma first blossomed, I joined monastics and lay friends in walking meditation, each step an invitation to arrive fully.

At Sarnath, also known as Deer Park, Thay gave a Dharma talk beside the Dhamek Stupa, marking the place where the Buddha first taught the Four Noble Truths and the Noble Eightfold Path. Listening to the living Dharma in that sacred space, the boundaries of time and place softened, and I felt the presence of my spiritual ancestors.

Visiting the sites I had so often read about brought the teachings vividly to life. We spent several days in Bodh Gaya, where Siddhartha Gautama sat beneath a bodhi tree and attained full enlightenment. A descendant of that original tree still grows there. We practiced sitting and walking meditation on the sacred grounds, where millions of pilgrims from around the world come to pay homage. The air is filled with chanting, and the collective energy is sublime.

Meditating beneath the wide branches of the tree, I felt the Buddha's presence—not merely as an abstract idea or even as Buddha nature, but as an intimate companionship, as if we were sitting together. My meditations are rarely cinematic, yet in that moment there was an unmistakable fullness. As I breathed in, I was surprised to notice a subtle, earthy, herbal scent. Without words, I asked for help in seeing as a buddha does.

We were sitting on a cushion of freshly cut kusha grass. As I rested there, my perception widened. What I had taken to be a simple bundle of grass began to reveal itself as a vast unfolding: water buffalo grazing downriver; flowering grasses; birds pecking through seed-filled dung and scattering them along the riverbanks. Sun, rain, and earth nourishing new shoots. Grass growing tall, spreading upriver, eventually harvested and bundled into this very cushion. And even now, in the fragrant, fresh-cut blades beneath me, I could see its future—drying, decaying, returning to the soil.

This realization came without words. Interbeing was no longer a teaching; it was fragrance, soil, and breath.

I understood then that to see like a buddha is to look beyond what we habitually recognize and name. With the Buddha eye, we look deeply to discern not only what is visible but also the vast web of conditions that precede and follow each manifestation. Every object, experience, and person arises through countless causes and conditions. We see mountain streams flowing through our veins and the same energy that moves the stars in our beating heart. A smile carries generations of healing; a single step holds both our ancestors and our aspirations for future peace.

When we cultivate the Buddha eye, we are no longer imprisoned by the illusion of separation. We touch the truth of interbeing and see that nothing exists independently; everything contains everything else. The discrete is no longer opposed to the whole. We look deeply and recognize the vastness—the great nature—within each apparent singularity. This understanding transcends our conditioned notions of same and different, self and other. It is captured beautifully in these words by Dr. Martin Luther King Jr.:

> *We are caught in an inescapable network of mutuality, tied in a single garment of destiny. Whatever affects one directly, affects all indirectly.**

Traffic is something we often contend with, perhaps something we dismiss as an annoyance. Yet when we investigate with the Buddha eye, its true nature, woven from countless causes and conditions, reveals itself: the invention of the wheel, fossil fuels, engines, roads, and the countless people whose lives intersect in

* Dr. Martin Luther King Jr., "Letter from Birmingham Jail," April 16, 1963, in *Why We Can't Wait* (Signet Classics, 2000), 87.

that moment. Our frustrations can become a mindfulness bell that invites us to pause, surrender, and recognize this moment as the crest of a wave, not random or separate, but arising from the sum total of our personal experience and the whole of human history. The traffic jam, the red light, and even our resistance are fruits of interbeing. We may not choose the wave, but we can surf it with awareness—or be pulled under by the riptide of habit energy. The choice, moment by moment, is ours.

When we approach life with curiosity and interest, investigation becomes a living practice of looking deeply. The koan "What is this?" invites us beyond surface appearances. We pause to explore the causes and conditions at play, both within us and around us. As we begin to see these patterns clearly, investigation becomes the insight that guides wise action.

## The Dharma Doors of Difficulty

Most of the Twelve Steps point us toward the shadow side, encouraging us to find a new way to engage with what troubles us. My practice community calls these growing edges—the ragged places where we get snagged offer real opportunities for growth.

In Step work and meditation, we turn inward to see things more clearly. Through the Dharma doors of powerlessness, resentment, shame, fear, shortcomings, and harms we have caused, we come to understand noble suffering. These cycles are known as samsara. Suffering sucks, but samsara is not separate from nirvana. Suffering is the ground of awakening. Without it, Siddhartha wouldn't have become the Buddha. None of us would have found our way to the freedom of recovery. Samsara and nirvana are two sides of one coin.

In Buddhist terms, ignorance is the root of suffering. Ignorance doesn't imply stupidity or a lack of intelligence. It means we are not seeing clearly. We have a wrong view. We cling to what cannot last and push away what we don't want, imagining ourselves as separate. Our grasping and aversion give rise to craving and a subtle yet persistent dissatisfaction, even in abundance.

We blame ourselves and others, getting lost in our stories and mistaking our interpretations for reality itself. We fall prey to countless forms of fear and live in confusion. But when we turn toward our confusion with mindful investigation—when we examine it closely rather than looking away—we discover it is fertile ground where insight can bloom. In recovery, this willingness to look deeply is exactly what Step Four asks of us.

## Looking Deeply: A Practice of Non-Fear

> **Step Four:** *We made a searching and fearless moral inventory of ourselves.*

When asked what meditation is, Thay would often reply that "meditation is taking the time to look deeply." That teaching resonates strongly with Step Four. I've come to appreciate the quiet depth of it. At first, it felt underwhelming. Brother Pháp Hải helped me touch the deeper meaning in Thay's words. He describes looking deeply as becoming intimate with the object of our attention. Looking deeply requires the willingness to meet our experience exactly as it is. This applies to meditation and the heart of Twelve-Step work.

In Step Four, we take the time to look deeply: to become intimate with what's blocking us. Through inventory, we investigate our thoughts, feelings, perceptions, and patterns of behavior. This isn't a ritual of blame or shame; it's a practice of clarity. With honest self inquiry, we begin to distinguish between what actually happened and the story we've told ourselves about it.

This fearless investigation is possible because we've already laid a strong foundation. With the stability of Step Two and the commitment of Step Three, we can turn toward our fears, resentments, shame, and hurts. Not to dwell on them, but to understand our wrong views and clarify our perceptions.

We examine our relationships, emotions, behaviors, and equally important, our strengths and assets. This work can be intense, even overwhelming, which is why it's essential to do it with the guidance of a sponsor or spiritual friend who has walked this path before.

When we investigate old memories and unresolved pain, we may find ourselves back in the emotional atmosphere of the past. This isn't a failure—it's part of the healing process. Healing occurs when we bring those younger parts of ourselves into the safety of the present moment, where we have resources, support, and perspective we didn't have before. In meetings, people sometimes say they're feeling angry, depressed, or irritable, then add with a knowing chuckle, "I'm writing an inventory." The room usually erupts in laughter and sighs of recognition.

In inventory, we put things on paper that we never expected to share with anyone. Writing down what we have long hidden is an act of non-fear. It is a liberation from wrong views and the distortions of self-protection. In doing so, we begin to forge new character traits and deepen our commitment to the path of recovery and awakening.

When someone does something that hurts us, our first instinct is to blame. They become the perpetrator; we cast ourselves as the victim. We interpret tone, words, or actions as personal attacks, even when none were intended. But one thing is certain: we are the ones who are disturbed. And that's good news. There's something we can work with.

Behind every resentment is a perceived hurt or threat. Instead of focusing on what they did, we can turn inward and ask: What in me is hurting or afraid? We set aside the mental replay and tend to the part of ourselves that's suffering right now. Our emotions become the object of investigation. We stop feeding the story and reconnect with what's alive in the present moment.

It's funny how we cling to resentments as if they were precious. "Do you know what so-and-so did?" We rehearse old conversations, imagining what we should have said. The Buddha named this dynamic more than 2,500 years ago with the teaching of the second arrow. When we experience pain, it's like being shot with an arrow. This first arrow, our initial hurt, is often unavoidable. The second arrow is self-inflicted: our reaction of blaming, ruminating, and feeling bitter. We are now victimizing ourselves, magnifying and prolonging the original pain.

I've become so skilled at shooting myself with a second arrow that I sometimes mistake it for happiness. With mindful investigation, I step out of the story and listen tenderly to what hurts, the way a good friend would. Rather than repressing or indulging these feelings, I discover that they're asking for something simple: to be seen, felt, and cared for. This is how the cycle of suffering begins to break: not by repressing or wallowing in emotion, but by meeting experience with mindfulness, curiosity, and compassion. We are responsible for our thoughts, words, and actions, but still powerless over what others may do.

Shame is one of the most insidious and pervasive emotions many of us carry. It's often said that resentment is the number one killer of an alcoholic or addict. I've come to believe shame is even deadlier, quietly fueling many resentments from the shadows. I am ashamed of shame and fearful of it, yet it, too, needs our loving care. Keeping secrets feeds shame; ignoring shame makes it stronger. It was many years into recovery before I could even name shame and longer still before I could sit with it tenderly in meditation. I learned to touch it tenderly and listen rather than run. It was a stroke of insight when I discovered that when shame arises, it doesn't mean I am shameful. It's simply a visitor; one we can meet with presence and care.

I revealed most of my secrets in my first inventory. Sharing the sexual ones took courage. It wasn't until the second or third inventory that I dropped the bomb: my deepest shame, the one that felt heaviest to name.

I admitted that I suffer from loneliness.

Loneliness has haunted much of my life.

Strong feelings like loneliness can be devastating. Its bodily sensation is the same across a lifetime. So it touches every moment we have felt it before. A moment of loneliness can swell into a tidal wave, threatening to drown me in a lifetime of isolation or pull me into a whirlpool of sadness or grief.

Emotions are more than mental states; they live in the body. When loneliness arises, I can feel it as a knot in the solar plexus, a heaviness in the chest, a hollowness in the belly. These sensations help me recognize and distinguish the emotion. Grounding awareness in the body allows me to meet the feeling directly and let go of the stories attached to it.

When strong emotions are seen, named, and lovingly held, they begin to loosen their grip. No words are needed. I hold the feeling in the arms of mindfulness—neither pushing it away nor clinging to it. I soften around the sensation and offer it compassionate companionship. I don't try to fix or erase the feeling; I simply stay present with it. When a feeling is met with embodied presence, the conditions for healing arise naturally, just as the breath deepens and slows with mindful awareness. Touching our pain with kindness, we discover a quiet resilience that doesn't force anything. We are no longer alone. We are fully with ourselves.

With mindfulness, gently guiding my attention toward what is healing and true, I can often recognize the smell and taste of loneliness as it begins to arise. I notice the stories that gather around it, the pull to spiral down into its vortex and dwell there.

Our emotions have Buddha nature: the capacity to change, heal, and reveal the truth. Each one is a precious, if sometimes well-disguised, Dharma door.

In the Fourth Step, we investigate the walls that confine us. The Fifth Step is a door to freedom and deeper healing.

## Stepping into Freedom

> **Step Five:** *We admitted to God, ourselves, and another human being the exact nature of our wrongs.*

In the Fifth Step, we share our written inventory with another person, typically our sponsor—a trusted elder in recovery. This step works on many levels. Some effects are immediate; others unfold more subtly over time. On the surface, this sharing deepens our Third Step commitment to the path. Writing a Fourth Step brings us into intimate contact with our shame, fear, trauma, and the ways we've caused or suffered harm. We list our resentments against people or institutions—the apparent objects of resentment—and then turn inward to discover the fear or wound that underlies each resentment. The hurt itself becomes the appropriate object of mindfulness.

The idea of sharing it all can feel paralyzing. Finishing the Fourth Step was a major milestone in my recovery, but calling my sponsor about the Fifth Step was a deeper surrender. I felt like I was hanging from a cliff, afraid to let go and trust another person with my secrets, shame, and fragility. I didn't like the way I had been, but comfort in the familiar held me back.

Experience shows that sitting on an unshared inventory is a recipe for disaster. It validates our fears and feeds our shame. It fortifies the walls of separation. Step Five is an act of faith in the recovery process. As Thay Pháp Lưu says, "We do not need faith in ourselves; we just need faith in the Dharma—confirmed by our own experience that it truly works." By the time we reach the Fifth Step, we've been around long enough to know the program is working, and we trust that it will continue to do so.

In the United States, "taking the Fifth" means staying silent. In recovery, taking the Fifth is an act of stepping into freedom. Sharing our inventory begins to dismantle the walls of isolation and transforms shame at its root. It challenges the old lie that we would be rejected if people knew who we "really" are. We long for intimacy, yet fear and shame often hold us back. When we believe those fears, we begin to doubt our goodness. This is the familiar terrain of imposter syndrome—the mistaken belief that our goodness is only a mask hiding our unworthiness. Little by little, we reinforce the lie that we are fundamentally damaged. If that's the case, what's the point of trying? Living in this way drove me toward substances.

When we share our inventory, fear and shame become connective tissue rather than barriers. In this surrender, the heart opens and softens. Our vulnerability is an expression of bodhicitta—the awakened mind of love that seeks healing for ourselves and for all who suffer.

Step Five is a practice of real community: showing up as we are and allowing ourselves to be held. Healing becomes possible in relationship; recovery is not a solitary path. It nourishes deep listening, truthful speech, shared insight, and mutual respect.

Reading our inventory aloud shifts our perspective. We hear our own words with fresh ears and see our patterns more clearly—both as participant and observer. Time itself adds perspective. When writing, we review the past from the present moment. By the time we read it aloud, time has passed. We meet the same words from a different place, with a different mind.

Seeing our story this way allows deeper understanding. We recognize patterns we once missed and see our role in past dynamics more clearly. The process reveals how fluid perception is, helping us reframe what we experience when familiar feelings arise again.

Awakening grows from the ground of fallibility and incompleteness. Wholeness isn't perfection; it's intimacy with our incompleteness. To be whole, we have to include all our parts.

Step Five marks a turning point. Our inventory shows who we have been; sharing it reveals who we are becoming. Grounded in honesty, humility, and willingness, we step more fully onto the path of recovery. It is a new beginning—a deepening connection to the program, to ourselves, and to the trusted friend who now knows us more intimately than anyone else. Built on courage and vulnerability, this relationship becomes a sacred support as we continue forward.

## Healing the Past in the Present

In the Fourth and Fifth Steps, I saw that some conclusions I came to as a child colored my worldview as an adult. Little Pete did his best to understand what was happening around him, but he reached conclusions without all the necessary information. Through Twelve-Step work and Thay's teachings, I've learned to be there for little Pete—to offer the love and understanding he never received.

Thich Nhat Hanh offered a meditation guiding us to see ourselves as a child, fragile, innocent, and vulnerable, and greet that child with a warm, loving smile. When I invite little Pete into the present moment, the heart softens with gratitude. He suffered greatly, but he survived. Sitting here with me now, he is safe. Together, we have wisdom and resources he never had. We can offer the care, protection, and compassion that we were denied growing up.

It is a marvel that so many of us survived the abuse, neglect, and unmet needs of childhood. After sitting with our five-year-old self, we can extend that compassion to our five-year-old mother, father, and siblings. This helped me understand their suffering. From a clenched heart, the flower of compassion blooms.

I used to resent my father. He was distant and emotionally unavailable. He didn't know how to play with me or even throw a ball. He was rigid, anxious, and didn't stand up to my mother. Seeing him as a five-year-old, I felt tenderness for little Dad. He never grieved the loss of his twin brother and grew up with a mother who told him the wrong twin had died. He never received the loving tenderness I longed for. Seeing him this way changed how I related to him as an adult.

When I feel anger or intolerance toward someone now, I sometimes invite them into my meditation as a five-year-old. This helps me cut through the story I tell myself about them. As children, we were all innocent, fragile, and shaped by the suffering around us. Some actions may be unforgivable, but looking deeply, we can recognize the wounded child and forgive the person without condoning the act.

I am learning how to care for and transform my trauma. When I am grounded, I can bring my younger self into the present, where he is safe, rather than reliving those hurts as a victim in the past. We can't change what happened, but we can change our relationship to it.

If trauma is passed from one generation to the next, so are resilience and healing. Our lives are part of a much larger unfolding. By transforming suffering in the present, we touch both the past and the future. We are healing our ancestors and descendants.

## A Healing Practice: Thích Nhat Hanh's Five-Year-Old Child Meditation

Find a comfortable posture and take a few moments to connect with your breath. If it helps you settle, place a hand on your heart or belly. Let your breath soften as you arrive in this moment. Relax and stay with each stanza until you feel connected before moving on.

*Seeing myself as a five-year-old child, I breathe in.*
*Smiling to the five-year-old child, I breathe out.*
*In: Myself at five years old*
*Out: Smiling*

*Welcome the child, care for them, share your peace and stability with them.*

*Seeing the five-year-old as fragile and vulnerable, I breathe in.*
*Smiling with love to the five-year-old in me, I breathe out.*

*In: Five-year-old fragile*
*Out: Smiling with love*

Touch their innocence with your heart. At that age, we are easily hurt. A harsh glance or reproachful word can wound deeply and give rise to shame. Our natural openness and trust feel unsafe when met with scorn. We learn to close down and harden our hearts. When we see ourselves as vulnerable children, compassion arises naturally. With a kind smile, we hold them in the arms of care. With love and gratitude, we honor their strength and endurance. Their resilience is now ours. Our safety and peace are now theirs.

You can continue by meditating on our parents as children. Begin with whichever parent feels easier:

*Seeing my mother/father as a five-year-old, I breathe in.*
*Smiling to my mother/father as a five-year-old, I breathe out.*
*In: Mother/father five years old*
*Out: Smiling*

*Seeing my five-year-old mother/father as fragile and vulnerable, I breathe in.*
*Smiling with love and understanding to my mother/father as a five-year-old, I breathe out.*
*In: Mother/father fragile and vulnerable*
*Out: Smiling with love and understanding*

We welcome the children who were our parents and smile to them as we would smile to a dear friend. Seeing their vulnerability, compassion is born, the meditation is bearing fruit. When we understand someone's suffering, acceptance and love naturally follow. Our resentments begin to soften.

*Seeing my mother/father in me, I breathe in.*
*Smiling to my mother/father in me, I breathe out.*
*In: Mother/father in me*
*Out: Smiling*

*Understanding the difficulties of my mother/father in me, I breathe in.*
*Determined to work for the release of both my mother/father and me, I breathe out.*
*In: Difficulties of mother/father in me.*
*Out: Releasing mother/father and me*

This meditation has helped me cultivate self-compassion and a genuine capacity for forgiveness. I have struggled with both. As you move through your day, try seeing the people you meet as five-year-olds, even for a moment. What changes when you see them that way?

## The Perfection of Aspiration

Having generated love and compassion for the five-year-old child, we can now extend that same care to our shortcomings.

> **Step Six:** *We were entirely ready to have God remove all these defects of character.*
>
> **Step Seven:** *We humbly asked Her to remove our shortcomings.*

After investigating our behaviors and relationships in Step Four and sharing what we've written in Step Five, patterns that cause suffering and block our spiritual growth begin to emerge. These ingrained behaviors—known as defects of character or shortcomings in Twelve-Step parlance—can be understood as habit energies: patterns of thought, feeling, and action that no longer serve us.

The language of Steps Six and Seven can be unsettling. Is our character really defective? Does healing actually require us to exile or erase parts of ourselves? Can deeply rooted traits truly be "removed" by effort, grace, or a higher power?

I worked these Steps as if my life depended on them. I examined each trait carefully—tracing its origins, questioning its purpose, and asking whether it still belonged in my life. This inquiry helped me become "entirely ready" to let them go. I humbly asked a higher power I didn't understand to remove them, and I felt a wave of freedom and lightness. Then, as often happens, these traits began to return.

In Buddhist language, our thoughts, speech, and actions are either skillful or not skillful. This framing is gentler and more compassionate than the language of defect and removal. What is unskillful isn't a fixed, separate entity that can be cut away. It is impermanent and conditioned—shaped by inheritance, environment, and habit—and therefore capable of transformation. The Buddhist path encourages us to recognize and embrace what is not yet skillful while clarifying and nourishing what is.

In both traditions, we turn toward what we would prefer to ignore. We investigate the behaviors we know are unhealthy but still cling to. The Buddha identified three core afflictions known as the three poisons: greed, anger, and delusion, sometimes called attachment, aversion, and ignorance.

Investigating the causes and conditions behind these behaviors, we often find fear at the root. When we exaggerate or embellish the truth, we may think we are enhancing our goodness. In reality, we are reinforcing the belief that we are not good enough as we are.

Willingness to change comes easily with some behaviors; others are sticky and seductive. I don't want to be a "complainer," but try going a whole day without complaining—it's harder than it seems. Then there's the familiar comfort of superiority and intolerance. Anger can feel justified, even empowering. And what about lust or sloth? There's a guilty pleasure in indulging them.

Digging deeper, I began to investigate the difference between pleasure and happiness. I discovered that living in alignment with my values brought a greater, more lasting joy than the fleeting pleasure of a bag of cookies or a moment of eye candy. As we work these Steps, we are invited beyond our comfort zone and our personal definitions of what is acceptable, toward our highest aspiration for human potential. This is an ever-deepening surrender that requires humility.

I experienced moments of absolute readiness—a feeling in my bones similar to the certainty I felt when I hit bottom.

At a deep level, I want to be the best person I can be: patient, understanding, and able to help others. I sincerely want to reduce the suffering I cause myself and those around me.

That desire to be free of afflictions is something pure and beautiful. The feeling of absolute readiness was fleeting, but I practiced cultivating it until it became familiar ground, a place I could return to. Once I could stand there with some steadiness, I moved on to Step Seven.

I wanted to believe that a divine power could simply eradicate my deeply ingrained patterns. But even with the sincerity of my best intentions, the shortcomings returned. At one point, I swore off Step Seven altogether, because the more I longed to be free of these traits, the more often they seemed to crop up.

In time, I saw this as a good thing. I had become more intimate with my habit energies. I began to recognize their cues and notice them before I acted on them.

Subtle changes in my breath and muscle tone warn me that anger is arising, and I can tend to it sooner. My nervous system still reacts, but I am better able to soften the intensity and shorten its duration. Old habits are persistent, like ruts our tires fall into, yet there is a way forward. With patience, clarity, and directed attention, we can gradually rewire our patterns of behavior.

Steps Six and Seven are aspirational. The moments of absolute readiness and willingness to live by our highest spiritual ideal are exalted states of liberation. The embodied aspiration itself is already complete, undiminished by the imperfection of our actions. Our humility refines and polishes the jewel of aspiration.

The Buddha offered medicine for our spiritual ailments. When he identified the three poisons, he also offered their antidotes: generosity, loving kindness, and wisdom:

| | |
|---|---|
| Greed | *Dāna* (Generosity) |
| Anger | *Mettā* (Loving Kindness) |
| Ignorance | *Prajñā* (Wisdom) |

This teaching informs my Seventh-Step practice. I no longer see defects as enemies to eliminate. They are misguided instincts, ignorant of the harm they cause—an invitation to love, not targets for eradication. My so-called defects are made of many wholesome elements. They, too, have Buddha nature and are part of the path to awakening. When I view shortcomings as "buddhas-to-be," they stop feeling defective and reveal themselves as assets in disguise. They are mindfulness bells, wake-up calls pointing toward growth. I see them as teachers, reminding me of the qualities I aspire to cultivate. This is spiritual alchemy: defects are not eradicated but transformed.

Thanks to impermanence, we have the capacity to grow and change. As skillfulness grows, what is not yet skillful is gently transformed. Our shortcomings become precious opportunities for practice.

## Tending the Garden of Mind

As we investigate the causes and conditions that shape our behavior, insight naturally arises. That insight ripens into discernment, revealing what leads to suffering and what leads to freedom. The idea of nourishing what is wholesome and not feeding the unwholesome may not sound like much of an epiphany. Yet this simple practice leads to and sustains the spiritual awakening that grows from Step work and looking deeply.

The Third Establishment of Mindfulness, mindfulness of mind, illuminates this beautifully. The guidance the Buddha offered is a way to investigate our mental states and discern which are helpful and which are not. He described these states as mental formations (Sanskrit: saṃskāra), because even what arises in the mind is shaped by causes and conditions. Nothing is fixed or permanent; everything can be understood and transformed.

The Buddha emphasized direct experience and careful investigation over blind adherence to doctrine. As a result, Buddhism is a living practice that continues to evolve. Centuries after his death, the Yogāçāra, or Mind Only school of Buddhist psychology, identified fifty-one mental formations. Eleven are considered beneficial, twenty-six unbeneficial or afflictive, and four indeterminate, depending on context. The remaining ten are considered neutral and universal.*

This may sound theoretical, but I've found it genuinely helpful in practice. The indeterminate formations loosen my rigid either-or thinking. For example, regret can be wholesome if it motivates skillful action, such as making amends, or unwholesome if it hardens into guilt or shame. Sustained thought can support investigation but becomes unskillful when it slips into rumination or obsession.

Mental formations are often described as seeds that remain dormant until they are watered. These seeds include mindfulness, compassion, joy, equanimity, and gratitude, as well as anxiety, anger, shame, fear, jealousy, and sadness. What a relief it was to discover that I am not defective or uniquely broken. These seeds are part of our shared human inheritance.

The dormant seeds reside in what is called store consciousness. Store consciousness holds these mental formations, along with everything we've experienced, perceived, or imagined. When conditions touch a seed, it sprouts and becomes active in mind consciousness. Thay often used the analogy of a basement and a living room: what appears in the living room is visible, while the basement holds what's out of sight. What arises in mind consciousness becomes the object of mindfulness in Steps Six and Seven and in the Third Establishment of Mindfulness.

---

* See appendix on page 187 for these fifty-one mental formations.

The more often a seed is watered, the more readily it sprouts again. Some seeds are conditioned by upbringing or inherited through family and culture; others are watered repeatedly by sense impressions. One seed can easily trigger another, setting off a chain reaction. For example, if I feel disrespected and react with anger, I might regret it later. Anger carries a toxic residue. On reflection, I may see that my reaction was unskillful, arising from seeds of hurt or fear. That recognition can water the seed of shame. If I'm not careful, my mind can spiral into self-obsession: What's wrong with me? My program and practice are a fraud.... In no time, the seeds of sadness, depression, or self-directed anger are watered as well.

With awareness and practice, I can water the seed of mindfulness when anger arises and step out of the spiral of self-obsession. With mindful presence, I am no longer caught in anger or its victim. I can breathe with it and care for it. This isn't an attempt to fix, suppress, or eliminate anger. It is being present with kind, compassionate care. As the renowned poet and teacher Stephen Levine said, "To heal is to touch with love that which was previously touched by fear."*

Our defects and shortcomings are impermanent. Through loving attention, we can hold them gently and gradually transform them, while selectively watering the seeds we wish to grow—kindness, acceptance, compassion, and understanding. Our beneficial mental formations are impermanent as well, which is why they must be continually nourished, as the Buddha taught in Right Effort.

The drawing that follows shows how Right Effort and mindfulness of mind work together. An unwholesome seed in store consciousness has become active in mind consciousness—let's call it anger. When it is recognized, the practitioner waters the seed of mindfulness to care for the anger, allowing it to settle and become dormant again.

---

* Stephen Levine, *A Gradual Awakening* (Anchor Books, 1979), 112.

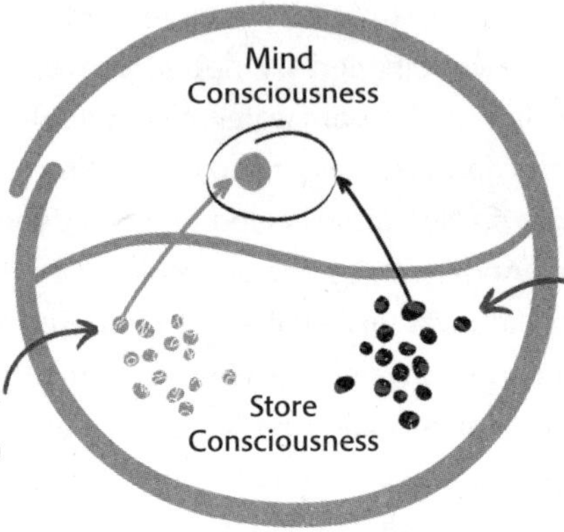


## Selective Watering

In the Plum Village tradition, the Yogācāra teaching of seeds and the Buddha's Right Effort come together in a practice known as selective watering. The gardening metaphor, which Thay often used, helps me practice with joy and ease. We feed and water what we want to grow, being careful not to nourish the weeds. Selective watering is a form of self-directed neuroplasticity. The seeds we water most often sprout faster and more vigorously. We replace old habitual responses with new neural pathways that support well-being.

This practice finds a clear expression in Right Speech, an element of the Noble Eightfold Path. Right Speech is abstaining from false, harsh, or divisive speech and idle chatter. Every word we speak waters seeds, wholesome or unwholesome, in ourselves and others. When we habitually express blame, anger, or intolerance, we strengthen those mental formations. Our inner dialogue, our thoughts and self-talk, matter too. When we practice loving speech, grounded in goodwill and compassion, we nourish those qualities and strengthen our aspiration.

Right Speech is a mindfulness practice not only in what we say but in how we say it. I've learned that my intention and impact don't always align. What is the kindest way to say this? Skillful speech grows out of deep listening. When I understand the other person's experience, I can shape my words so they have the best chance of being understood and well received. To harmonize my speech, I need to listen to the tone of the person I'm speaking with. Like music, timing matters too. Instead of speaking impulsively, I pause to consider whether they are ready to receive what I have to say. Practicing Right Speech requires diligence and care, which brings us to the Third Factor of Awakening.

# PART II

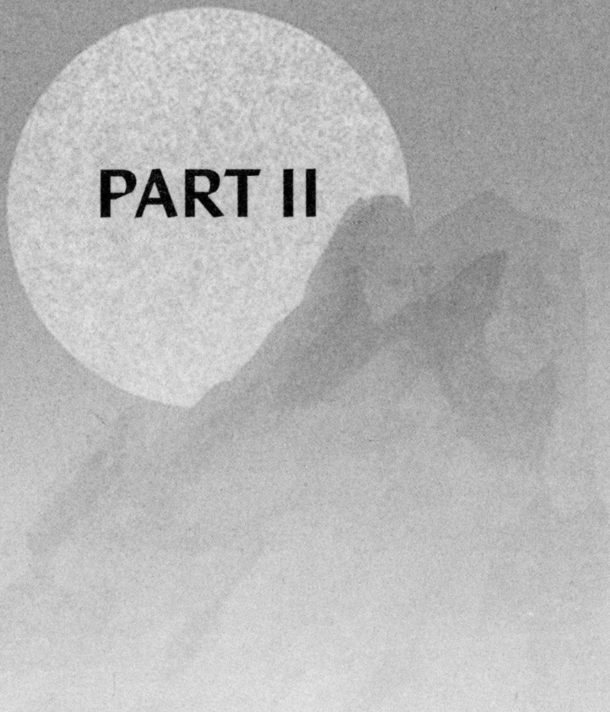

# Dwelling in the Refuge

## THE THIRD FACTOR OF AWAKENING:

# Diligence

*Vīrya* is generally rendered as diligence, energy, or effort, but these translations can miss some nuance. It also suggests enthusiastic perseverance. It grows from aspiration and confidence in the path, supported by mindfulness and investigation. The joy of well-being gives rise to this kind of perseverance.

## Living by Vow

The Buddha offered the Five Precepts for lay practitioners to support ethical living, designed to protect both the individual and the community from harm. The precepts guide us to refrain from killing, stealing, sexual misconduct, false speech, and intoxicants. After decades of study and practice, Thich Nhat Hanh offered a contemporary expression of these teachings called the Five Mindfulness Trainings.*

In Thay's words, "The Five Mindfulness Trainings represent the Buddhist vision for a global spirituality and ethic." Born of deep insight and compassion, the Trainings invite us to examine our actions, deepen our understanding, and cultivate conduct that reduces harm. They point toward the insight of interbeing—the lived understanding that our well-being is inseparable from the well-being of all.

---

* See appendix.

## Reverence for Life

The Buddha's first precept, non-killing, seems straightforward. Thay's First Mindfulness Training, Reverence for Life, plumbs the depth of this commitment. We vow to look closely at violence and compassion—not only in action but in thought, consumption, and habit. We consider how our daily choices contribute to harm or healing.

When I first encountered the Trainings, I still ate meat and thought I was entitled to do so. I dismissed concerns about environmental impact and animal suffering, numbing myself to the violence embedded in industrial food systems. We vow to take a more compassionate approach, one that was not entirely new to me.

As a teenager, inspired by a book about Gandhi, I had become a vegetarian. I cared deeply about animals and didn't want them to suffer. At sixteen, while staying with a family in Chiapas, Mexico, chicken was served in my honor. In broken Spanish, I explained that I didn't eat meat. My host family looked crestfallen and offered it again. When I declined a second time, their hurt and disappointment were palpable as they said, "We killed our chicken for you." I vividly remember the moment. My stomach dropped, and I felt untethered, as if I were floating above my body. I sensed their hurt and pushed it away. Feeling numb, I declined again.

I had compassion for the chicken, but I didn't consider my hosts.

Years later, I learned that the Buddha and his monastics ate whatever was offered during alms rounds. If it was meat, they accepted it, honoring the spirit of generosity. Compassion without wisdom can become self-righteous; wisdom without compassion can become cold.

The First Training has helped me cultivate a more nuanced compassion. Applied Buddhism can be sticky business. Some harm is inevitable, even with a plant-based diet. The intention is not purity or perfection. The commitment is to reduce the harm we cause.

I began with meatless Mondays, which grew into several days a week. I felt lighter and more intentional, in body and mind. Eventually, I became vegan, knowing it was still imperfect but less harmful than industrial meat production. Living by vow continues to deepen my aspiration as a peacemaker.

During a period of serious illness and grueling medical treatment, I became addicted to video games. The games I favored were first-person shooters. Over time, they numbed me to violence and conditioned me toward hyper-reactivity. That is a useful skill for gamers, but it left me jumpy and irritable when I stepped away from the screen. I began to see this as killing in the mind—and a form of intoxication.

During this same period, a close friend was dying of cancer, treasuring every remaining moment of her life. With the guidance of the Trainings, I let go of gaming and was inspired to live with greater presence and intention.

## True Happiness

In the Second Mindfulness Training Thay reframed the Buddha's second precept, non-stealing, as true happiness. We make a commitment to recognize the abundance already present. Happiness is not found in getting or becoming but in coming home to what is here.

Consumer culture trains us to believe happiness lies just beyond reach. It blurs the distinction between needs and wants. Online shopping can be incredibly addictive for me. Am I enhancing my life or trying to fill an imaginary void? Living from a sense of lack leads to grasping and clinging—a subtle form of self-victimization. With appropriate attention, we rediscover a wealth already ours: recovery, community, friendship, this breath, and the extraordinary woven into the ordinary. As gratitude grows, the restless hunger of wanting begins to settle. This is true happiness.

## True Love

Thay reframes the third precept on sexual misconduct as true love. We commit to a deeper practice of generosity and care.

There was a time when I used others for sexual gratification. It didn't matter whether they were in relationships or married; sex was another fix. It seemed to soothe my loneliness but only briefly. My hunger was rooted in greed—my needs eclipsed everything else. True love transforms that hunger into care for others. It nourishes connection rather than consumption, generosity rather than grasping.

This Training points to the four elements of true love: loving kindness, compassion, joy, and equanimity. Two of these—joy and equanimity—are also Factors of Awakening.

## Loving Speech and Deep Listening

The Buddha's fourth precept, refraining from false speech, is expressed in the Fourth Mindfulness Training as loving speech and deep listening. We commit to look deeply at how we communicate. Are my words true? Are they intended to heal or to harm? Do they nourish understanding or deepen division?

Grief has sharpened my sense of urgency around speech. I want to tell people what I appreciate about them while I can. I want to be as present with them as I wish I had been with David, my stepson. Speaking from the heart and listening deeply require spaciousness and care.

For years, I longed to speak privately with Thay—to tell him how much the practice had changed my life. When the moment finally came, nothing needed to be said. Bowing to one another was a complete transmission.

This Training remains a growing edge for me. I still swear reflexively at times, and though I enjoy colorful language, it's not always appropriate. I continue to work with unkind self-talk as well. These are trainings, not achievements.

## Nourishment and Healing

The Buddha's fifth precept is abstaining from intoxicants. Thay frames it as nourishment and healing. Those in recovery know abstinence is only the beginning. Without intoxicants, we're left with untreated addiction. Healing comes from untangling inner knots and caring for suffering instead of numbing it. In this training we examine everything we consume: food, media, conversations, and activities. What am I feeding in myself? What am I nourishing in others?

I modeled gaming addiction for young David, and that realization humbled me deeply. I've also come to understand gambling as profoundly intoxicating. It has harmed many people in recovery and their families. What once felt like harmless social fun proved otherwise. I no longer participate. I want my actions to preserve peace and well-being.

## Receiving the Trainings

I practiced the Five Mindfulness Trainings for some time before formally receiving them. The transmission ceremony connects us to an ancestral stream: a gift of Dharma handed down from the Buddha through generations of teachers and practitioners. This mirrors Twelve-Step recovery, where the path is passed down from sponsors to sponsees. Receiving the Trainings was a commitment to live by vow, much like the Third Step.

On October 28, 2008, I received transmission of the Five Mindfulness Trainings and the Three Jewels from Thich Nhat Hanh on Vulture Peak. I was given the lineage name Deep Transformation of the Heart and was honored to join the Lam Tế (Lin-ji) and Liễu Quán Dharma lineages.

# Reconciliation: Turning the Wheel of Karma

Karma is a Sanskrit word meaning "action," which includes the results of what we do. As the Buddha taught, karma includes thoughts and speech as well as bodily actions. Karma operates according to cause and effect: our actions leave traces that create conditions for what will come to be.

In recovery, we begin to see how our past actions shaped our present: the wreckage we created and the relationships we damaged. Through the inner work of the Steps—especially Four through Seven—we come to understand the patterns that shaped our past. But insight alone is not enough. Steps Eight and Nine are where insight becomes action and we turn toward those we have harmed.

> **Step Eight:** *We made a list of all persons we had harmed and became willing to make amends to them all.*
>
> **Step Nine:** *We made direct amends to such people wherever possible, except when to do so would injure them or others.*

When we acknowledge the harms we've caused and take responsibility for them, making a sincere effort to repair the damage, we turn the wheel of karma from ignorance toward understanding and reconciliation. Making amends is an act born of humility and a profound Dharma door that opens to freedom for ourselves and those we have harmed.

The process of reconciliation begins within. As we look honestly at the harms we've caused, our inner landscape becomes clearer. We uncover the fear, confusion, and habit energy that shaped our actions and begin to soften toward the wounded parts of ourselves. This clarity is inner reconciliation: coming home to the truth of who we have been and who we are becoming.

Our understanding and healing give rise to bodhicitta, the awakened heart that wants to relieve suffering and repair harm. Bodhicitta gives us the energy to make amends, not from guilt or obligation, but from understanding and love. We step forward as peacemakers, committed to living with care, connection, and ethical conduct.

In Step Eight, we examine how our actions have affected others emotionally and materially. This is a different kind of inventory, and we approach it with Right Intention, nourishing recovery rather than shame. At this stage, the work is solely for our own clarity. We set aside thoughts of Step Nine and give our full attention to understanding the impact of our actions. With mindfulness of body, feelings, and mind, we hold the weight of what we've done with care for ourselves and those we have harmed. Becoming intimate with the karmic residue of our actions begins the process of atonement—"at-one-ment."

For a time, I practiced with the Zen Peacemakers tradition and chanted the Gatha of Atonement, translated by Roshi Taizan Maezumi:

> *All evil karma ever committed by me since of old*
> *on account of my beginningless greed, anger, and ignorance*
> *born of my body, mouth, and mind*
> *now I atone for it all*

Chanting and reflecting on this gatha deepened my understanding of the Eighth Step and widened its application. Having looked deeply into my personal life, I began to investigate ancestral and systemic harms. Many of the comforts I take for granted are built on suffering. I live in California, on land that was taken from Indigenous peoples and from Mexico. My home sits on a hillside where native species have been displaced. As a white American, I benefit from a dominant culture shaped by violence, oppression, and slavery. As a man, I receive wages, opportunities, and privileges that are not equally available to many women and people of color. I'm not responsible for creating all of these conditions, but I am responsible for recognizing injustice and working to transform the systemic conditions that deny and sustain harm.

Even language carries karma. Phrases like "master bedroom" trace back to histories of slavery and plantations. The Mindfulness Trainings are a practice of looking deeply—not to feed shame but to grow awareness. Exploring male privilege and the imprint of patriarchy has been challenging and illuminating. I am not responsible for the advantages I inherited, but I am responsible for how I respond to them. I care enough to cultivate awareness and use my privilege for the benefit of all beings.

I struggle when reading the news because it is so disturbing. I limit my exposure but refuse to turn a blind eye to what's happening in the world. Isn't it appropriate to be disturbed by violence, greed, and injustice? At the same time, vigilance is important. I protect my resilience so I don't burn out and can respond with wisdom.

I abhor racism and intolerance so much that I become intolerant of it. My outrage can feel justified, but any intolerance is the same poison. How do I reject cruelty and violence without dehumanizing the perpetrators? Hating the haters is still hate. I need both heart and mind to keep my compassion alive and find the Middle Path between indifference and obsession. I can't change the world overnight, but I trust that every act of kindness moves us in that direction.

What if everything we complained about disappeared?
"Ugh, is this person sharing again?" Poof—they're gone.
"My dog's barking again—I wish he'd stop." Poof—no dog.
"I wish Mom didn't have dementia." Poof—no mom.
Poof—no me.

## Living Amends

Atonement begins as an inner shift and finds its fulfillment in action. The willingness to make amends in the Ninth Step comes from a change of heart. I justified my harmful actions by pointing to other people's behavior. With awareness, that defense fell away. My pain—in the form of shame and regret—became a bridge to the pain I had caused others. My heart softened with compassion. This was our pain. There was no spiritual justification for it.

My parents were at the top of my amends list. I had stolen money and precious objects; I had lied to and manipulated them; I had caused a world of hurt, fear, and disappointment. They were mortified when the police knocked on their door looking for me, embarrassed when friends asked how I was doing, and broken-hearted not knowing where I was, living or dead. In the later years, their fear for me became fear of me. After supporting me through therapy, detoxes, and treatment programs, they eventually cut me off and told me I was no longer welcome.

Months later, horribly addicted and scuffling for cash, it occurred to me that the huge record collection I'd left at their house was worth a good chunk of money. I called and asked if I could come by. My father met me at the door with a shotgun. He was terrified of me. This was a doctor committed to saving lives, pointing a deadly weapon at his son. I was clearly drug crazed and denied entry. I waited on the porch while he and my brother Jeff brought the records out. I never spared a thought for them. All I could think about was the next fix.

How do you make amends for that? Or make amends for not being the son they needed when their eldest son, my brother Richard, took his life? For becoming another source of suffering—another absence—status unknown. Expressing remorse and making financial restitution began the process of reconciliation, but paying back the money and expressing regret was a bandage over a deeper wound. How do you restore trust? Repairing the emotional and psychological impact of my actions required time and a sustained change in behavior, something words alone could never accomplish. The real amends are lived and expressed in all future actions.

When I went to my parents' house to make amends, we were all nervous and uncomfortable. For the first time, I didn't need to convince them I was clean. They could see it in my eyes and demeanor. I wanted nothing from them. I was making amends for my own freedom and to protect my recovery. They listened. It was a beginning.

We had become strangers. I tried to see them with fresh eyes and let go of old resentments and disappointments. As an ongoing amend, I committed to visiting every other week for at least fifteen minutes. It wasn't easy. I remember sitting in my car at the curb, praying to a god I didn't believe in for the courage to walk to the door. Over time, I added phone calls on the alternate weeks and took an interest in their lives. I was diligent. This was my living amends.

Gradually, our relationship changed. One day, I leaned in to hug my father—a natural expression of connection. He stiffened. Hugs weren't part of our family culture. I explained that it was something we do in recovery, and that made it acceptable. In active addiction, we spread dysfunction. In recovery, we send out ripples of healing. In the truth of interbeing, my recovery was mutually healing. On my next visit, my father greeted me with a hug. It became something we both looked forward to.

I was breaking the cycle of samsara by offering what I had always longed for and never received. I no longer blamed my parents for their shortcomings. I felt compassion for them—for the love they themselves never received. We often think the past is gone and unchangeable, but it lives on in the present moment. When we meet it with understanding, we can transform the past in the present.

Decades later, my father developed Alzheimer's, and there were many challenges. I lived a hundred miles away but did my best to support them both emotionally and spiritually. Alzheimer's is often hardest on the caregiver. In time, my mother reached the point of surrender. When she told me she could no longer live with him, I was judgmental. I came to understand that his decline was heartbreaking for her, and his care was more than she could manage.

I moved my father to San Diego and became his guardian. It was a burden of responsibility, but I was honored that my mother and brother trusted me with his care. I could do what they could not. There were many moments of love, surrender, and insight. It broke my heart every time I bought adult diapers for a man who had once been a meticulously clean physician. When the time came, I was entrusted with the decision to move him into hospice care. I am profoundly grateful I was with him the night he died—holding his hand, telling him it was okay to let go, that his work was done, and we were all cared for.

When I left that night, I felt grief and unexpected peace. I had lived my amends through his final breath. My recovery was truly lived in every fiber of my being.

A decade later, I cared for my mother as I had cared for my father. She developed dementia, and though her decline was painful to witness, our relationship was tender and loving. She often said she had lived a wonderful life and was ready to go. She asked me not to replace her pacemaker battery when it ran out. When it malfunctioned, I declined the doctor's offer to replace it. It was one of the hardest decisions I've ever made, but I honored her request as a final act of loving kindness. My wife and I were with her, holding her hand as she took her final breath. There was sadness but no regret.

Living our amends is more than cleaning up the past. It's a commitment not to cause that harm again. We transform our karma, using the harm we've caused as fuel for awakening. Consequences may continue, but from this point forward, we are defined by who we are becoming, not by who we were.

I continue my Ninth Step work through what we call indirect amends: service, giving, and advocacy for peace and justice. I vow to honor those I have harmed, along with my parents, teachers, and ancestors, by calling on the Medicine Buddha to help me bring relief from suffering, in myself and in the world.

## Beginning Anew

*In true dialog, both parties are willing to change.*

—THÍCH NHAT HANH

It's said that wherever two or more gather, conflict is inevitable. Sister Chan Khong and the Plum Village community developed a practice called Beginning Anew to restore harmony and healthy communication. As the name suggests, it is a practice of renewal—turning toward connection as medicine for separation—and a mindfulness practice grounded in loving speech and deep listening. In the formal ceremony, only one person speaks at a time. A vase of flowers is often used as a "talking piece" to make this clear.

The practice has four parts: flower watering, expressing regrets, sharing a hurt, and sharing a long-term difficulty and asking for support. Usually, the first two restore harmony; the third and fourth are used when deeper healing is needed.

### Part One: Flower Watering

Flower watering is a practice of appreciation. We reflect on the qualities we genuinely admire in the other person, often naming specific examples so our appreciation is grounded and real.

Being angry or hurt does not erase another's goodness. We set grievances aside and practice appropriate attention, allowing ourselves to see what is good and beautiful. When I do this sincerely, my perception often shifts. My heart softens, and relief naturally arises.

Grief has taught me to water flowers regularly. I train my mind to notice what is good in others and express sincere appreciation while I still can, even if it makes me feel vulnerable. I also take joy in watering the flowers of strangers. If I notice a kindness—from a receptionist, a waiter, or a passerby—I say so. A caring word brightens both our days.

We all long to be seen and valued. I carry childhood wounds around feeling invisible, which can make receiving praise uncomfortable. I tend to deflect or joke to avoid that tender vulnerability. When my flowers are being watered, I practice mindful breathing and allow the words to land in body and mind. When negative self-talk arises, I return to my breath and ground in mindfulness of the body, letting appreciation land. It is not a moment for deflection or correction—only listening.

## Part Two: Expressing Regrets

Expressing regrets resonates with the Eighth and Ninth Steps of recovery. This practice blends the Dharma's wisdom on reconciliation with the program's emphasis on amends. Apologies can feel hollow. But when we mindfully hold a feeling of regret for what we've said, done, or neglected, that sincerity is alive in us. Our words carry humility and vulnerability. This vulnerability helps the other person soften. Connection is restored.

## Part Three: Sharing a Hurt

Sharing a hurt is a practice of nonviolent communication grounded in loving speech. We speak honestly, not destructively, with the intention of restoring harmony. In emotionally charged situations, a neutral person can help. Often, it's wise to practice sitting or walking meditation beforehand to care for seeds of anger or reactivity. Mindful breathing calms the body, which in turn calms the mind and emotions. From that steadiness, peacemaking can guide us.

When listening to a hurt, we do not interrupt. Letting go of right and wrong, true and false, we listen with compassion, holding the intention to relieve the other person's suffering. No response is required except regret. This is not the time to explain or defend. Even if we believe the other person has misunderstood us, we thank them and reflect on their words. If needed, we can schedule another Beginning Anew where we are heard.

### Part Four: Sharing a Long-Term Difficulty & Asking for Support

At times, old wounds resurface in the present, causing real difficulty. When we share our struggles honestly, others can know us more deeply. Understanding our challenges allows others to support us.

## Righting a Wrong View

Some amends unfold on their own timeline.

In 1982, after returning to California from New York City, I reconnected with Laurie, a high school friend. We hit it off right away and shared a fun, affectionate relationship. Before long, we were living together. I was getting high recreationally but was off narcotics, and it felt like a new beginning.

Almost a year later, Laurie became seriously ill with intense cramping. When she passed out the next morning, I called an ambulance. At the hospital, she was diagnosed with an ectopic pregnancy. The fetus, lodged in her fallopian tube, had grown large enough to rupture it. She was bleeding internally and would have died without treatment.

When she was released a few days later, her mother insisted she recuperate at her home. Within a week, Laurie unexpectedly broke up with me. She never explained why.

I was devastated. Convinced it was my fault, I concluded that I was fundamentally unlovable. My hopes for a new life collapsed, and I sank into shame, despair, and active addiction. My life unraveled until I hit bottom a few years later.

When I got clean, I inventoried the relationship. Even off narcotics, I saw that drugs were still central to my life during the time we shared. Laurie never complained, but I had hidden parts of my drug use. Being stoned created a fog between us, whether she consciously recognized it or not. I also believed drugs kept me from showing up with real presence when she was rushed to the hospital. Laurie went onto my Eighth Step list, and I felt it was important to make amends.

She remained on my amends list for decades. I tried to find her periodically, before and after the internet, but without success. Her mother was also on my list; I had burglarized her home a year after the breakup. I remained willing to make amends when possible and considered my sobriety an indirect amends until something changed. It was the best I could do.

In 2021, a mutual friend wrote asking if I was the same Peter Kuhn who had once been with Laurie. She had read an article about my recovery and renewed music career and was seeking support for her addicted son. When we spoke, Gloria mentioned Laurie was happily married and living in New England. She added that Laurie had always spoken kindly of me, which confused me after so many years of relentless self-blame. I told Gloria I wanted to make amends, if Laurie was willing, and asked her to pass along my information.

A year later, Laurie left a friendly voicemail on my birthday. I took a day to reflect on the amends I wanted to make before returning her call. At first, I assumed it was about addiction. Looking more deeply, I realized Laurie had known about my history and accepted it. What I regretted, perhaps sharpened by David's death, was not having been more emotionally available or offering the support she deserved. I wanted her to know I had worked on this over the years and now strive to show up with wholehearted presence in my own marriage.

When I called Laurie back, my intention was to clear my side of the street. We talked at length. She told me I had been kind, caring, and present during our time together. She remembered me staying up with her all night before we called the ambulance. She said she never fully understood why she broke up with me.

I finally saw that the end of our relationship was shaped by many conditions—not a single cause. Not just me. The near-death experience was severe trauma, compounded by an unexpected pregnancy and the loss of the baby. When I mentioned my own trauma work, Laurie said she didn't believe she'd experienced trauma. I gently pointed out that she had nearly died from internal bleeding and was rushed to the hospital. She paused, then said she had never thought of it that way but could see it now. We both recognized we were young and living in a time with little awareness of trauma.

As we spoke, something became clear. It wasn't just "a tubal pregnancy." The embryo that almost killed her was our baby—my only child and hers. I had been oblivious to this grief for decades. A mix of wonder and sorrow arose. I touched my own grief while helping Laurie care for hers.

Understanding the role trauma played in our breakup was revelatory. It allowed me to reexamine decades of suffering through a new lens. Not everything that affects me is about me.

My wrong view of the breakup led to years of suffering. Convinced of my inherent unworthiness, I took responsibility for forces beyond my control. I reached conclusions without all the information and lived in ignorance for decades. Learning to recognize and care for these old hurts, rather than believe them, is the substance of my practice and recovery. As Stephen Levine often said, it is "the healing I took birth for."

## Polishing the Gem

Even those of us who stay engaged in recovery and practice go through periods when focus fades and enthusiasm wanes. Staying motivated on a spiritual path can be challenging. Our minds are pulled in a thousand directions, and meetings or meditation can begin to feel like chores rather than nourishment. Understanding the inner energies that guide us helps sustain what we most want to grow.

Volition is the inner force that moves us forward. Aspiration is the heart's deepest desire, the north star that guides us. Diligence is the energy that keeps our actions aligned with our values. When our thoughts and actions are in harmony with our aspiration, practice can take on a devotional quality, bringing a subtle joy and reverence. Recovery and insight naturally flourish. This brings us to Step Ten and the practice of daily inventory.

> **Step Ten:** *We continued to take personal inventory and, when we were wrong, promptly admitted it.*

We are taught to work the Steps in order, but we don't leave one behind as we move to the next; we carry them with us. The Steps are composite, like all dharmas. Steps One through Nine are woven into Step Ten. In Step Ten, we continue the practice of mindful investigation, shining the light of recovery on the familiar sources of suffering identified earlier: fear, anger, resentment, shame, blame, and other behaviors that are not yet skillful. We may ask: Where have I been unskillful, self-centered, or reactive? Where have I contributed to conflict? What needs acknowledgment or correction?

Pema Chödrön offers a helpful reflection for the end of the day:

> *At the end of the day, before going to sleep, think over what you've done. If you fulfilled your aspiration, even once, rejoice in that. If you went against your aspiration, rejoice that you are able to see what you did and are no longer living in ignorance. This way you will be inspired to go forward with increasing clarity, confidence, and compassion.**

For me, what began as an evening review gradually flowed into my day. I became more aware of my motives and the character of my thoughts, words, and actions.

---

* Pema Chödrön, *The Pocket Pema Chödrön* (Shambhala, 2008), 59.

Being mindful of the body helps me recognize when I'm tense or upset. Being mindful of feelings reveals what I'm resisting or clinging to. Being mindful of the mind helps me understand the seeds I'm watering. When the unconscious thought "What's in it for me?" becomes conscious, it may soften to "How can I help?"

At Plum Village practice centers, mindfulness bells are an essential part of daily life. Whenever a bell sounds before meals or during activities, or even when a clock chimes, we pause, return to our breath, and come home to ourselves in the present moment. Even a ringtone can become a mindfulness bell. Mindfulness is heartfulness; each pause restores presence.

Mindfulness bell apps are available.* I have Twelve-Step sponsees who don't meditate but use the bell as a reminder to pause and pray during the day. It's a simple way to bring practice into busy lives. Stopping for the bell isn't always convenient. The sound reminds me to live by vow, heartfully, with kindness and care.

As practice deepens, we cause less harm, and our Tenth-Step reflections become more nuanced. We are always practicing something: What am I practicing in this moment? Is my behavior aligned with the amends I made in Step Nine? Am I still committed to transforming the unskillfulness that Steps Six and Seven focus on? What supports my growth? What does not?

One of Thay's questions was, "Am I sure?" It asks us to investigate our perceptions. Am I sure of this person's intention? Am I sure they're a jerk? Am I really listening—or just hearing? Am I listening with the ears of my heart?

Thay and the Buddha were often repetitive. At times, I'd catch myself tuning out when Thay told a familiar story—until I noticed my reaction. Am I sure I don't need to hear this again? Am I sure there's nothing more to learn?

---

* The Plum Village app includes a programmable mindfulness bell along with talks, meditations, and study resources.

The Sutra on the Eight Realizations of Great Beings was one of Thay's favorites. Brother Pháp Hải shared that he found it dull and sat through years of recitations with his eyes closed. Decades later, he fell in love with it, discovering it contained the entire wisdom of the Buddha. His book, *The Eight Realizations of Great Beings*,* is a masterpiece. Our sangha studied it for years, and we continue to practice with it.

Our peace, joy, and compassion are revolutionary. If we were on a small boat, lost at sea without food or water, and it sprang a leak, how would we want to meet that moment—sharing fear and panic or with a steady presence, a small smile from a life well lived, and a warm, compassionate hand on someone's shoulder? Death is inevitable; how we meet it is not. Every moment is precious, never to return. May we live each one with love and integrity.

I use Thay's "Gatha on Impermanence" as a daily Tenth-Step reflection. It helps polish the gem of my aspiration.

> *This day is ending; our lives are shorter.*
> *Let us look carefully at what we have done.*
> *Let us practice diligently, putting our whole heart into the path of awakening.*
> *Let us live deeply in each moment,*
> *free from our afflictions and aware of impermanence,*
> *so that life does not drift away meaninglessly.*

## Everyday Zen

Words matter. The phrase "worked the Steps" can suggest completion, as if they were a one-time assignment to be checked off. Some approaches to recovery treat them that way, but I was taught differently. The Steps are not finished; they are metabolized. They

* Brother Pháp Hải, *The Eight Realizations of Great Beings: Essential Buddhist Wisdom for Waking Up to Who You Are* (Parallax Press, 2021).

shape how we see and engage with the world. We continue to surrender, take inventory, make amends, deepen our conscious contact, and apply these principles in our lives. We work the Steps forward, backward, and inside out, using them as a compass.

Thay's teachings are offered in the same spirit. As a novice monk, Thay's first assignment was to memorize short verses called *gathas* to support mindfulness in daily activities. There are gathas for turning on a light, following the breath, brushing your teeth, or using the toilet. They are silently recited, one line with the in-breath and the next with the out-breath, inviting a pause to stop and touch presence. When I got Thay's book *Present Moment, Wonderful Moment,** I posted gathas throughout the house as mindfulness bells. I've shared a few of my favorites below.

I cannot overstate the value of gatha practice. Gathas have profoundly deepened my practice and the quality of my attention. I spent much of my life sleepwalking on autopilot. Gathas remind me that every moment is a potential awakening. Every breath and action can reveal a poem or a song, a chance to touch the sacred.

These gathas are small practices for daily life. They are meant to be revisited with the breath, not completed. When we allow the shift to happen, they awaken presence and reveal the gift of each moment.

### Waking Up

*Waking up this morning, I smile.*
*Twenty-four brand new hours are before me.*
*I vow to live fully in each moment,*
*And view all beings with eyes of compassion.*

I recite this before getting out of bed and feel spiritually awake.

---

* Thich Nhat Hanh, *Present Moment, Wonderful Moment: Verses for Daily Living*, 3rd ed. (Parallax Press, 2022).

When David died, I understood how precious our moments are. The vow to live fully in each one brought me to practice. As I silently recite this in the morning, I renew that aspiration. To live fully in each moment is to live in mindfulness. My heart opens as I vow to view all beings with eyes of compassion, and I remember that includes me.

I turn on the water tap without thinking—water flows from the faucet, nothing special, right? When I am truly present, the miracles of ordinary moments are revealed.

**Turning on the Water**

*Water flows from high in the mountains.*
*Water runs deep in the Earth.*
*Miraculously, water comes to us,*
*and sustains all life.*

This gatha reminds me that water is precious. Not everyone has access to clean water. As I visualize snowcaps feeding mountain streams and rivers, I feel refreshed and connected to nature. I remember that the Earth holds water beneath the surface, just as my body does.

These verses connect me to Thay and our spiritual ancestors. Gathas remind me that every moment holds awakening.

When I look in the mirror, I judge what I see and call "me." Do I look good or bad, neat or messy, tired or fresh? With the mirror gatha, something shifts:

**Looking in the Mirror**

*Awareness is a mirror,*
*reflecting the four elements.*
*Beauty is a heart that generates love,*
*and a mind that is open.*

Reciting these lines, I pause and ask: What is doing the seeing? Awareness reveals itself, distinct from thought. Looking deeply, I cultivate Right View and touch my composite nature. I am made of water, air, minerals, and the play of energy. I am woven from the elements of mountains, rivers, and stars.

What I call "me" is a miraculous gathering of trillions of cells, organs, and nonhuman life—microbiota that sustain this body. Even my appearance is not mine. It is inherited through countless generations. The face in the mirror carries my ancestors.

Breathing with these verses, my fixation on appearance softens. I touch a deeper reality. Thoughts, words, and actions are our true belongings. "Beauty is a heart that generates love and a mind that is open." With this gatha, I step beyond conventional labels and touch the ultimate nature of reality.

As an improvising musician, I hope to live with that same creative fluidity. When I am fully present, all is music. My music embraces every sound an instrument can make, including squeaks, squeals, honks, and wails. Music reflects the times we live in.

I want my music to carry morning light and birdsong, as well as the cries of injustice, fires, floods, and violence. It holds the joy of reconciliation, the harmony of kindred spirits, and the wonder of being alive. We play sound and silence.

The Buddha embodied skillful means, adapting his teachings to meet each being where they were. There are stories of him calming a charging elephant with nothing but his presence. Music is universal; plants and animals respond. Our words are music, like birdsong. May they carry freedom and joy.

Gathas help us return when attention slips. Diligence is not always long periods of meditation; sometimes it's the willingness to pause and begin again. And again. Many happy returns.

## THE FOURTH FACTOR OF AWAKENING:

# Joy

The Buddha's teachings were transmitted orally for hundreds of years before they were written down. He taught in the language of his time, and they were later preserved in Pāli and Sanskrit. As we know, words carry worlds within them, shaped by the meanings we inherit and reinforce. Ancient terms don't always map neatly onto modern English, and something can be lost in translation.

As we move into joy, translation matters again. In the Pāli texts, *pīti* is often rendered as rapture or bliss—words that can sound dramatic or otherworldly to Western ears. Some descriptions speak of a bright energy moving through the body as the mind focuses.

In Sanskrit, the same quality appears as *prīti*, often translated as joy or delight. This points to something more familiar and accessible. Joy grows from mindfulness, curiosity, and care. When we meet experience with gentle interest, the heart begins to brighten.

Joy is a byproduct of alignment; it's not an achievement reserved for advanced meditators. In the Plum Village tradition, joy is nourished as an everyday medicine, available to anyone who can breathe and touch the present moment. If there is no joy in our practice and recovery, it will not be sustainable. It is a companion on the path, not a reward at the end.

In the Ānāpānasati Sutta—the Buddha's discourse on mindfulness of breathing—there is a clear distinction between joy (pīti) and happiness (*sukha*). Joy rises like a wave as the mind clears; happiness rests like a calm shore. Thay offered this image: "When you are crossing a desert and out of water, seeing an oasis ahead is joy. When you drink the water, that is happiness."

What does joy feel like in your body and mind?

Rising or buoyant energy?

Lightness in the breath?

Warmth in the chest or belly?

Spaciousness, cooling, tingling, or ease?

When joy arises, practice mindfulness of the body. Make a home in the feeling. Become intimate with it.

Small joys appear every day, but we often treat them as drive-bys—acknowledged with a passing thought as we rush to the next distraction—rather than stopping to feel them. The feeling of joy is the same, whether it comes from a blade of grass pushing through a sidewalk or a surprise visit from a loved one. When we pause to absorb these sensations, fleeting joy can become more sustained. Over time, these moments become a resource we can return to and draw upon to refresh our resilience.

Gil Fronsdal, a noted Buddhist scholar and teacher, suggests that joy is a feeling of affirmation:

> *Yes—to the breath.*
>
> *Yes—to this moment.*
>
> *Yes—to being fully present.*
>
> *Yes—to the body, to the sensations, to the truth of experience.*
>
> *Yes—to opening to the joy that comes from non-conflict with the moment.**

## Joy, Happiness, and Pleasure

If joy is so available in the breath and in small moments, why do we miss it so often? Part of the answer is how we understand joy, happiness, and pleasure.

---

* Gil Fronsdal, "The Power of Yes," talk given at Insight Meditation Center, Redwood City, CA, October 3, 2011.

In the Buddha's teachings, joy and happiness are distinct but related. Joy has an uplifting, energizing quality—like a fresh breeze in the heart—while happiness is quieter and steadier. Both are part of the path and can be cultivated.

We tend to use these words interchangeably, but our ideas about them can get in the way of actually experiencing them. As the Dalai Lama reminds us, "Remember that sometimes not getting what you want is a wonderful stroke of luck." There is joy in recognizing that the absence of a toothache is a kind of happiness.

As an addict, I was a relentless pleasure seeker. I confused it with happiness. But as Brother Pháp Hải says, "It's like licking honey off a razor blade." Pleasure is sensory, dependent on conditions, and fleeting; it easily leads to craving and clinging. Happiness is an inner state of well-being, less dependent on circumstances and nourished by living in alignment with our values.

I learned this the hard way. I was afraid to go to Twelve-Step meetings, yet they brought joy and freedom I never imagined. At first, I was reluctant to go to Deer Park Monastery, and later unsure about committing to a Buddhist tradition. Feeding fear shuts the door on joy and happiness. Finding a teacher who spoke to my heart and a community aligned with my aspiration and values brought benefits I never could have predicted. To touch the joy of awakening, I had to free myself from the fears that would have paralyzed me.

After practicing the Five Mindfulness Trainings, I felt called to go deeper. I expressed my aspiration to ordain and spent years being mentored as an aspirant to the Order of Interbeing. In this period, my aspiration deepened and became clearer. I trained in ethical conduct and the forms of practice and facilitation, learning how to honor my teacher and our lineage. In 2010, I received the Fourteen Mindfulness Trainings and was ordained by Thich Nhat Hanh at his monastery in France.

At ordination, we are given a Dharma name. I received the name Chân Hỷ Hải, True Ocean of Joy. I was taken aback. I had suffered so deeply that I thought there had been a mistake. Me—an ocean of joy? I had been an ocean of suffering, shaped by fear, loneliness, addiction, crime, incarceration, and trauma. I had caused great harm. What were they thinking? I came to see that joy is not the absence of suffering but the capacity to care for it and shine light in the darkness. The elders saw what I could not: the ocean of joy is as deep as the ocean of suffering. How could it be otherwise? They recognized joy in my aspiration and my willingness to serve the dying, the incarcerated, and those seeking recovery. It didn't mean I was carefree or frivolously happy. The joy they saw was my commitment to the path and to loving service.

## Both/And

We've seen that joy can be found in what is present and what is absent. When things go wrong, we can still touch and nourish joy. Brother Phap Dung, a Dharma elder who encouraged me to write this book, shared the story of a child who dropped a plate of food during eating meditation at the monastery. Eating meditation is a reverent time, a silent practice of collective mindfulness. When the plate shattered in the silence, a jarring wave of sound swept through the room. You know what that's like. The crash is startling, even in a busy restaurant.

The child froze. The parents jumped up, mortified, rushing to clean up the mess. Brother Phap Dung knelt beside the young one and invited a pause. Smiling, he said, "Look at how beautiful the colors and patterns are on the floor. It's like art." There is beauty in the mess when we look with loving eyes. In the same way, there is joy and unexpected beauty in the messes of our lives, if we pause, breathe, and smile.

Is there joy in the death of my seventeen-year-old stepson? I still remember the tidal wave of sensations: the floor dropping away, my stomach falling, my throat tightening, my breath caught in cold disbelief. When I think of David with love and tenderness, tears still rise. The wrongness of it, the injustice of a young life ending so abruptly, still stirs anger and grief. Yet there is joy in remembering the happiness he knew: his music, his laughter, his playful spirit, and the many ways his life touched mine. He loved the color orange, and my heart still lifts when I see that bright, generous hue.

One day he brought home a tiny gopher snake. Caring for it planted something unexpected in me and remained part of my life long after David's passing. In Zen, we speak of "both and." Joy and sorrow are not opposites. The heart is not binary. People cry at weddings and sometimes laugh at memorials. David's death changed my life in utterly devastating and profoundly formative ways. In a real sense, his death became a rebirth for me. Heart-breaking and unmistakably a gift.

We can bring this spirit into the ordinary moments—even a meal. There is joy and suffering in the food before us. Eating meditation helps us hold this reverent awareness.

## Eating Meditation

Eating meditation begins with mindfulness of the meal and the food before us. Though I share here the practice of eating meditation in community, you can also enjoy a mindful meal in solitude. In community, it begins with silence, followed by mindful conversation. We practice being joyfully present with one another and with the food. We begin by bowing to our empty plate and reciting the following gatha:

> *My plate, empty now, will soon be filled with precious food.*
> *Beings all over the Earth are struggling to live.*
> *How fortunate we are to have enough to eat.* *

---

* Thich Nhat Hanh, *Present Moment, Wonderful Moment: Verses for Daily Living*, 3rd ed. (Parallax Press, 2022).

Seeing the coming into being and dissolution of the kusha grass cushion at Bodh Gaya has stayed with me and given me new eyes. Thanks to impermanence, everything we take to be solid is continuously transforming. Eating meditation helps us see with the eyes of interbeing, looking beyond the labels we habitually use, and touching true nature. We share a smile with those around us and, with palms together at the heart, recite:

> *This food is a gift of the earth, the sky, numerous living beings, and much hard and loving work.*
>
> *May we eat with mindfulness and gratitude so as to be worthy to receive this food.*
>
> *May we recognize and transform unwholesome mental formations, especially our greed, and learn to eat with moderation.*
>
> *May we keep our compassion alive by eating in such a way that reduces the suffering of living beings, stops contributing to climate change, and heals and preserves our precious planet.*
>
> *We accept this food so that we may nurture our brotherhood and sisterhood, build our Sangha, and nourish our ideal of serving all living beings.*

The first contemplation invites awareness of the countless causes and conditions that brought this food to our plate. It cultivates Right View and a living connection with the earth. The second invites mindfulness of the food and our companions. Some stumble over the phrase "worthy to receive." It doesn't imply unworthiness. It invites us to receive the meal with humility, honoring the natural forces and human labor that made it possible. This humility supports spiritual growth.

The third invites eating in the spirit of the Middle Way. We become attentive to greed and excess, eating slowly and with care. As the saying goes, "Drink your solids and chew your liquids."

Every bite is sacred. We take only what we need, eating for nourishment and nourishing appreciation. How many bites do we truly taste? The first bite can be heavenly, and then the force of habit takes over. I often catch myself loading the next forkful or thinking about seconds before I've finished what I have. When I eat mindfully, I rest the fork between bites and fully receive each one.

The fourth contemplation brings our food choices into the light of compassion. We look honestly at how our meals affect other beings and the planet. Plant-based diets can significantly reduce environmental harm and the suffering embedded in industrial food systems. The fifth nourishes our aspiration not only to eat for ourselves but to benefit all beings and to use the energy we receive to live with Right Action.

These contemplations come before eating for a reason. Once we begin, we remain present rather than lost in thought. There is joy in noticing the colors, shapes, flavors, and textures of each bite. We can see the sun, rain, and earth in our food.

Food arrives as something we experience as "other." Digestion begins as saliva and teeth break it down. As we swallow, it is already becoming us. What was other becomes blood, bone, muscle, and energy. The body's wisdom is astonishing: without conscious effort, it extracts what is needed and releases what is not. What we once considered delicious eventually becomes something we call waste.

Toilet meditation may sound humorous, yet it is a profound Dharma door drawn from the Heart Sutra (Prajñāpāramitā Sūtra). It invites us to let go of our notions and see each moment as the ground of awakening.

### Using the Toilet

*Defiled or immaculate,*
*increasing or decreasing—*
*these concepts exist only in our mind.*
*The reality of interbeing is unsurpassed.*

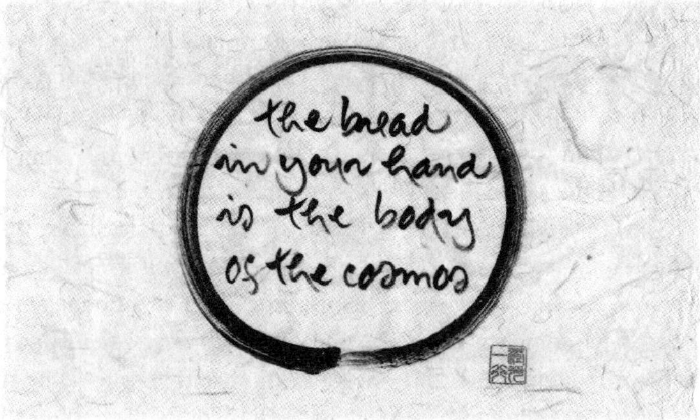
the bread
in your hand
is the body
of the cosmos

Thanks to impermanence, what the body releases continues transforming. Composting returns nutrients to the soil and grows more food. What we call a meal is only a moment in a vast, intimate cycle. When we see eating clearly, we touch interbeing. We are not separate from the earth. We are the earth.

## Boundless Love

I loved and appreciated David while he was alive. We had our difficult moments, but he was a bright, beautiful spirit. After his death, I found myself dwelling on what I missed. They say grief is love with nowhere to go. At first, love fed my grief and intensified the loss. I called on my love to nourish despair, confusing the intensity of the feeling with a kind of closeness. Eventually, I realized the David I grieved would want me to be happy rather than sorrowful. Long, painful mourning wasn't honoring the goodness of the life and love we shared. What honored him was my joy, my laughter, and my passion for life.

But grief kept calling. Between moments of reprieve, it returned—raw and forceful. I think of grief as a spiked meat tenderizer, not to pulverize the heart but to soften it. Is there a "right" way to grieve? I have friends who lost a beloved pet and vowed never to get another. They said the pain was too much to bear. I've learned to lean into it.

Love is both noun and verb. As a noun, it's a feeling. As a verb, it's an action. Breathing in, love is present. Breathing out, I smile. When I shine the light of love on an object of mind, it reveals love—even in sorrow. I vow to soften my heart around grief and never get over it.

Grief contains non-grief elements. What feels like a dark, bottomless pit is the shadow cast by the light of love. Sitting with grief, I learned to care for it rather than dread it or feel victimized by it. The more I practice love as action, the more my capacity to love expands. I became able to love what I once thought unlovable.

In mourning David, I came to see that grief is layered and pervasive. We grieve the loss of drugs when we stop using. We grieve the job we didn't get, the one we lost, the end of a marriage, the death of a friend. Grief is connective. When it arises, it rarely comes alone; it awakens echoes of every loss we've known, touching all our tender places.

In the years after David's death, I often drove to the tide pools in Point Loma. At times, I felt like I was drowning in an ocean of sorrow, alone in a bubble while the world carried on, indifferent to my devastation. He was a surfer, and sitting at the intersection of ocean and land helped me open to a broader perspective.

There was a veterans' cemetery on the way, and I usually drove past it without a thought. One day, passing row after row of identical white headstones, something shifted. The markers weren't scenery. Each one was a life. Someone's child. Someone loved. The headstones multiplied my grief beyond measure, echoing my loss back to me.

Gazing at those anonymous graves, I realized the grief I swam in was not mine alone. An uncountable number of parents, partners, and friends were touched by loss, unseen companions in a vast field of shared sorrow.

The reality of our shared grief hit with visceral force. This wasn't mine; it was ours. A moment later, even that dissolved. It became grief without object, no longer mine, theirs, or ours, but universal, inseparable from love, timeless and without identity.

Love is not fixed or possessed. It is composite, made of countless elements: my mother's love, David's love, the kindness of teachers and friends, the tenderness of strangers, the presence of the sacred. My heart opened as what once felt like separation became connection. If I can no longer share my love with David in physical form, I can share it with others, with life itself. This embodied love needs no object for validation. It is love without borders—a boundless force of nature.

## Objects of Mind

Seeing that my love for David could be directed to others revealed something important about how the mind works. It always has a focus. It is always relating to something. Addiction isn't only about substances. It reflects the mind's tendency to grasp—what we experience as obsession, craving, and compulsion. When we get clean, the mind looks for something else to attach to. Gambling, food, sex, work, exercise, politics, or even spiritual seeking can become new compulsions.

The Buddha spoke directly to this pattern in the Fourth Establishment of Mindfulness: objects of mind. The pattern of obsession remains even as the object changes. When we become mindful of what we're fixated on, we can pause, breathe, and gently investigate: What am I really craving? Is this worthy of my energy and attention? With awareness, we may see we long for belonging or connection; the object we cling to may only be a stand-in. Freedom begins with this insight.

When I'm aggravated, everything is aggravating; objects for my irritation are endless. When I'm steady and grounded, sources of joy are just as abundant. With Right Mindfulness and Right

Effort, everyone and everything, including our irritation, can become an object of awakening. Turning toward the experience of irritation rather than its object is the path of healing. This is the same movement we make in inventory, when we look within at the resentment itself rather than focusing on who we resent or what happened. We can loosen our internal knots, but remain powerless over the objects: people, places, and things.

My joy in the Dharma has deepened my joy in recovery, just as my joy in recovery has deepened my joy in the Dharma. With the eyes of mindfulness, there are said to be 84,000 Dharma doors.* One can easily substitute recovery for Dharma in this verse from the Dhammapada, a collection of the Buddha's early teachings:

*The gift of Dhamma surpasses all gifts.*
*The taste of Dhamma surpasses all tastes.*
*The delight in Dhamma surpasses all delights.*
*The destruction of craving conquers all suffering.*

—DHAMMAPADA 354

The two paths are not merely compatible; they are mutually regenerative—intertwined and ever-nourishing.

## Joyfully Letting Go

In Twelve-Step meetings, they said, "The only thing you need to change is everything." I wasn't sure what that meant, but doing recovery on my terms hadn't worked. I needed to do things differently. So when I came back to the program this time, I made the difficult decision to step away from playing music. Playing in clubs and bars felt like a setup for relapse, and I needed to "square up." That meant getting a day job, paying rent, and becoming a

* In early Mahayana texts, 84,000 represents an immeasurable, inconceivably large number of teachings and methods.

responsible member of society. At the time, that was changing just about everything. It was a profound surrender, but I was willing to do whatever it took to stay clean. That meant changing everything: my lifestyle and ideas about what was hip and what was square.

The Pete who got me to the rooms of recovery had little to offer when it came to living in recovery. I rarely spoke about my life as a musician and focused on the life I was building. That strategy served me well. There was no inner conflict, just a steady commitment to the path I had chosen.

The surrenders kept coming. When I was five years clean, I stopped smoking cigarettes. I could have said the self-destructive addiction was no longer aligned with my values, and that would have been true. But it wasn't quite enough to let go. I kept getting chest infections and knew smoking was part of the problem. That weighed on me. What finally shifted things was a casual comment from a supermarket cashier.

In those days, you could smoke anywhere. Standing in line at the market one day, impatient and frazzled, I had a salty attitude and probably made it known. I felt entitled and indignant; the person ahead of me was taking too long in the express lane. As I loaded my groceries for the cashier, I had a cigarette dangling from my mouth. Ash fell on the counter in front of her, and I shrugged. She looked up as she rang up my items and said, "I hate people who think the world is their ashtray."

I'd never considered that, but it was true. I flicked ashes and cigarette butts wherever I pleased. I emptied my car's ashtray into the street without a thought. I cared about the world, and this comment stopped me short.

I've struggled with my weight and body image for most of my life. Maybe it's genetic or my addict nature—but I love eating. Countless diets left me feeling tormented, fixated on what I was missing. As Carl Jung observed, "What we resist persists." Eating meditation and mindful consumption offered an approach that felt harmonious and supportive rather than punitive. Like abstinence, they required a shift in perception born of surrender. With mindful consumption, not eating the cookie can bring greater happiness than the brief pleasure of eating it. What once felt like restriction now feels like freedom. It was the same when I stopped eating meat: a joyful choice, an expression of care rather than deprivation. Over time, I've learned that joy often lives on the other side of release.

> *If by renouncing a lesser happiness*
> *one may realize a greater happiness,*
> *let the wise one renounce the lesser,*
> *having regard for the greater.*
>
> —DHAMMAPADA 21.290

My work was going well. I was selling semiconductors and proud to be supporting my family. My manhood was tied to my income, and I became obsessed with money, property, and the prestige of being a top salesperson. It became an identity—a mask I hid behind—with the mistaken belief that success and happiness were the same thing. One day, a handwriting expert offered free readings at a local bookstore. After looking at my writing, he said, "I see you're not happy in your work."

I laughed and straightened him out right away. "Sorry, you've got that one wrong. I'm making big bucks, and I'm at the top of the company in sales."

He smiled and replied, "I didn't question your success. I said you weren't happy."

I couldn't hear him at the time. I was convinced success was happiness. A few years later, I was fired, and everything changed. I had been sick with liver disease, made worse by the devastating side effects of treatments I had hoped would cure it. Without my job, I felt lost and rudderless. Who was I now?

Most of us pass through these dark nights of the soul. As the Reverend Dr. Martin Luther King Jr. said, "Only when it is dark enough can you see the stars."

My life took an unexpected turn. I became a professional reptile breeder known as Python Pete. Inspired by David, who brought home the baby snake, I ended up with a house full of rare pythons. I realized that like a snake shedding its skin, I had to let go of my image as a high-powered professional.

I had mistaken that image for proof of recovery.

Working with snakes produced a happiness that had been missing in my old job. I built one of the first reptile websites, connected with a global community, and supported our family for years without missing a beat.

## A Gift in the Wound

Impermanence never stops. Does that make it permanent?

My liver illness progressed, and in time, I could no longer manage the reptile business. I was struggling on the meds, dealing with anger and depression. My wife and I drifted apart after twenty years of marriage. I sat with the dynamics between us, our growing disconnection, and took inventory of my actions and inactions. We tried counseling and made sincere efforts to reconnect, but it felt irreconcilable. As it became clear that many of the forces at play were beyond my influence, accepting that our marriage had become unmanageable took time. Old tapes of unworthiness and inadequacy played softly in the background: Was this a failure of my recovery or practice? If I were stronger, could I fix this?

My practice of compassion still had room to grow. I'd worked hard to understand my wife's suffering, but I hadn't offered the same compassion to myself. Before we married, I had promised myself I wouldn't be the one to quit. I had to reexamine that vow.

Each of us deserves a partner who understands and appreciates us as we are. Living with constant strain was unhealthy for both of us. When I asked whether she wanted to continue or part ways, she chose divorce. Love, in this case, meant letting go.

In the spirit of surrender, my heart's wish was freedom for us both, whatever that looked like. I trusted we would each find the happiness we deserved. What if nothing needed to be fixed? After all, every bond is subject to change, whether we're ready for it or not. There was relief, and even joy, in the clarity of letting go.

After our divorce, loneliness and grief haunted the space my wife had occupied. Returning to the basics of Twelve-Step wisdom, I attended a meeting or practiced with my sangha daily. One night, shortly after she moved out, a group of us stayed for nearly an hour after the meeting: we laughed, talked, and enjoyed each other's company. I drove home feeling light and connected. As I approached the house, I noticed the porch light was off. There was no one there to turn it on. The house felt dark and unwelcoming.

Inside, it felt cavernous. What had once been filled with the sounds of children and family was now silent. After twenty years of living with others, it was shocking to be alone. In the bedroom, I saw the king-sized bed we'd bought together, now half empty. I turned on the TV. It was a show we had always watched together. When I heard the theme music, a heaviness settled in. I turned off the TV as a wave of loneliness hit me.

Years of practice had prepared me for moments like this. I returned to my breath. *Breathing in, I know loneliness is here. Breathing out, I am here for you, my loneliness.* I stayed with the sensations—the weight in my solar plexus, the hollow in my belly. Loneliness felt familiar, almost timeless. It whispered, "You were lonely before you met her, and you are lonely now. I'm here to stay." I breathed with it like a mother cradling a crying child, neither resisting nor feeding it. I watched it arise, remain, and pass. I acknowledged what was true: yes, loneliness had been present before, and yes, it was here now. But it was also true that just an hour earlier I had been laughing with friends, connected and alive. *Dear loneliness, you come and go like passing clouds. I am here for you; not all is loneliness.*

Feelings arise unbidden but not without a cause; a sound, a song, a season can call them forth. Whether they become poison or medicine depends on how we relate to them. Feelings are real, but the stories we attach to them are not. The feeling of loneliness didn't disappear, but my relationship to it changed.

As I continued breathing, I noticed a story attached itself to the emotion: "You're lonely because she's gone. You blew it. If only she were here, everything would be okay." With each breath, I offered compassion to the ache. Clarity arose: getting her back was not the answer. I had been lonely even while we were together. I didn't need her—or anything outside of me—to be okay.

Wanting to honor the grief and the love I felt, I decided not to date for a year. It was a gift to myself: time to grieve, to look deeply at what I truly wanted in a partner, and to avoid rushing into another relationship out of loneliness.

A few days later, still tender, I went to an evening meeting with a friend. During the break, I stepped into the bathroom. As I stood at the urinal, I silently recited my version of the toilet gatha:

> *Standing solid on the ground, I smile and release.*
> *Water comes to me and through me, sustaining all life.*

As I began to urinate, I had a delightful insight: there was no grief or regret in letting go. The water had once been nourishing and life-sustaining, but now my body released it freely, without clinging. Fresh water quenches thirst, but passing it is also a joy.

Though the child in me felt rejected and abandoned, another part of me felt grateful for the twenty-two years we shared. We supported each other through some of life's hardest moments. By any measure of the heart, our marriage was meaningful. It was the longest committed relationship of my life, and I learned about love, care, and showing up.

In the months that followed, I came home to myself and rediscovered that I am enough. It was a restoration to wholeness, and being single brought unexpected joy. A soul song stirred.

THE FIFTH FACTOR OF AWAKENING:

# Ease

## Effort and Ease

The pithy slogans that once hung on meeting-room walls are less common in the meetings I attend these days, but their spirit remains alive. *One Day at a Time, First Things First, Keep It Simple*—these reminders point to appropriate attention: keeping recovery and sobriety primary. *One Day at a Time* is the heart of Twelve-Step wisdom. We don't have to stop forever; we just take care of today. It's the same in mindfulness; we take it breath by breath. Caring for the present creates the conditions for the future.

*Easy Does It* may be the most iconic slogan, recognized both inside and outside the rooms of recovery. I saw it on bumper stickers long before I understood its meaning. When I came into the program, people said, "Stop and smell the roses." I took this expression to mean "Show up for life with more joy and ease." Thay said essentially the same thing: "Walk as if your feet are kissing the earth," and "Smile to your breath." Different traditions, different words, same wisdom.

The importance of ease—the settling of body and mind as effort is released—is foundational in Buddhist teachings on mindfulness meditation, particularly in the Satipaṭṭhāna Sutta (The Four Establishments of Mindfulness) and the Ānāpānasati Sutta (Mindfulness of Breathing). Both offer detailed guidance that begins with calming the body, allowing ease to arise naturally.

## In/Out, Deep/Slow Meditation

Meditation is mind training. We learn to distinguish between thought and awareness. Awareness is the stable, receptive field in which thoughts arise. Attention is awareness with direction. In meditation, we guide attention rather than trying to control thinking. Guiding attention isn't mind over matter or mind dominating mind. Trying to think our way into silence is like yelling, "Quiet," in an echo chamber.

Meditation is profound surrender, a shift from habitual thinking to direct awareness. The shift is subtle but monumental. As I move through the day, I pause to ask, "Am I really present?" I am when the extraordinary is revealed in the ordinary, when every breath is a source of joy.

Meditating with a goal is a recipe for frustration. Program literature speaks of quieting the mind. I took that literally and thought it meant silencing my thoughts. Trying to will the mind into silence tied me in knots. Thinking generates more thinking. Quieting the mind is better understood as calming the mind. The Buddha used that language in the Sutra on Full Awareness of Breathing. By bringing attention to the body—to breathing, heartbeat, sensation, or contact—thoughts recede into the background. We don't push them away; we allow them to settle. Ease comes from nonresistance.

We cultivate stillness, but it is not absolute. Blood moves through the body, the heart beats, and as the earth spins at a thousand miles per hour, we move with it. Quieting the mind is also relative.

I tried to cultivate a daily meditation practice for years, but it never took root. That changed when I found *Be Free Where You Are* while visiting Deer Park Monastery after David's death.* Thay

---

* Thich Nhat Hanh, *Be Free Where You Are* (Parallax Press, 2002).

shares a deceptively simple meditation based on the Buddha's teachings that remains the foundation of my practice. I wrote the following verses down and kept them by my meditation cushion, practicing with them until they were deep in my bones:

*In/Out*
*Deep/Slow*
*Calm/Ease*
*Smile/Release*
*Present Moment/Wonderful Moment*

Breathing with the first pair of words, silently acknowledge "in" with the inhale and "out" with the exhale. Mindfulness of breathing begins with mere recognition: *Breathing in I know I am breathing in; breathing out, I know I am breathing out.* Mind and body come together as we touch what is real and true in the present moment. We're not thinking about the breath. Our attention rests in the sensation of this very in-breath and out-breath.

## In, Out

As our attention settles on the breath, our breathing smooths without conscious effort. We may notice the in-breath deepen and the out-breath lengthen as a natural result of our attention. When this happens, we move on to the next pair of words:

*Inhaling, we silently say "deep."*
*Exhaling, we gently say "slow."*
*Deep . . . slow.*

As mindfulness becomes steady and sustained, we can stay with the whole breath from beginning to end. Our attention is focused and concentrated. We enjoy breathing. The in-breath gives rise to the out-breath; the out-breath completes and fades—impermanence in action. As the body and breath become calm, the mind follows. We calm the mind by calming the body. When there is calm, ease naturally arises.

*Breathing in, we acknowledge calm.*
*Breathing out, we nourish ease.*
*Calm, ease.*

We stay with each phrase until it feels real and true. If it doesn't, we return to the previous verse until the next naturally unfolds. Calm and ease aren't imposed; they're rediscovered.

When body and mind come into harmony, it feels good. Enjoying that goodness, we smile.

*Breathing in, I smile.*
*Breathing out, I release.*
*Smile . . . release.*

The body and breath are always in the present moment, and when mind and body are together, we are truly here—stable and solid in the now. Breathing in, we silently say "present moment." Breathing out, we acknowledge the joy of our breathing and sitting. This is a "wonderful moment."

*Breathing in, present moment.*
*Breathing out, wonderful moment.*
*Present moment, wonderful moment.*

In recovery and meditation, we learn to meet and accept ourselves just as we are. When thoughts race, we acknowledge them with kindness and compassion: "Breathing in, I know my thoughts are racing; breathing out, I smile." This is mindfulness of mind: awareness calms what it touches. By returning attention again and again to the breath, we learn to rest in awareness, no longer victims of our inner weather. We are more than our thoughts.

The Chinese character for mindfulness (念) is composed of two elements. The top (今) signifies now; the bottom (心) is translated as heart/mind. Buddhist mindfulness is more than being in the present moment. It is heartfulness, experienced as friendly care, curiosity, joy, and ease.

Missing a day of practice isn't failure. Noticing is mindfulness. Our regret means we care. We can nurture that care instead of turning it into shame.

If I forget to sit for meditation before leaving home, I pull over and sit for a bit in my car. Even a few minutes make a difference. When meditation feels like a chore, I've forgotten the joy of sitting and turned it into labor. I sit in an easy chair instead of on a cushion and keep it short. Anyone can sit for three minutes. When the pressure lifts, joy returns. I usually feel so good I remember why I like it and want to sit longer. With mindfulness, every breath affirms our worthiness.

## Working Meditation

In the Plum Village tradition, effort is always paired with ease. Everything is a meditation, including work. This is different from our usual work world, where getting things done often matters more than how we do them. In working meditation, we do not push to get a task done; we enjoy each moment, usually in silence, without hurrying or worrying. Our work is a loving service to the community, and our mindful presence and care are as much a gift as the results of the task.

Work periods are an opportunity to build community and often begin with practice songs, which are themselves a meditation. The lyrics are Dharma teachings set to simple melodies—easy to remember, deep enough to guide us. As we sing, we are invited to embody the words, allowing them to settle into us (and sometimes to arise later, like seeds sprouting after rain). There is a spirit of playful joy in the singing that we carry into the work. One song that speaks to this spirit of ease is "And When I

Rise," a folk song by Wendy Tuck, adapting a poem by Wendell Berry:

> *And when I rise, let me rise*
> *like a bird, joyfully.*
> *And when I fall, let me fall,*
> *like a leaf, gracefully, without regrets.*
> *And when I stand, let me stand,*
> *like a tree, strong and tall.*
> *And when I lie, let me lie,*
> *like a lake, peacefully, calm and still.*
> *And when I work, let me work,*
> *like a bee, wholeheartedly.*
> *And when I play, let me play,*
> *like a breeze, refreshingly, light and clear.**

Working meditation has changed the way I approach everyday tasks. I sometimes guide prison inmates through the Steps by mail when no local sponsor is available. I've also written to people who reach out to Plum Village monasteries seeking support while incarcerated.

Sometimes important activities feel like busy work. I've learned to wait until I have the space to answer these letters with mindful care. When I notice myself hurrying, addressing envelopes while already thinking about what comes next, that urge to finish becomes a mindfulness bell. Aware of my freedom and of where these words are traveling, I place each stamp with tenderness.

I am easily swept into busyness and can forget that each moment is equally precious. On the clock at work, we may think freedom comes at the end of the day. But every moment is our time,

---

* "And When I Rise," *Basket of Plums Songbook*, ed. Joseph Emet (Parallax Press, 2013), 27.

never to come again. We can reclaim our freedom with every mindful breath.

## Lazy Days

The image of a bee moving lazily from flower to flower as it collects pollen for the hive is a treasure. Yet "busy as a bee" is a familiar saying, and laziness is often an accusation that carries moral judgment. Maybe buzzing lazily is how bees manage to work so tirelessly?

Working meditation and lazy days are two sides of the same coin. In the first, we learn to show up wholeheartedly, with joy, whatever we are doing. In the second, we affirm that our worth does not depend on productivity.

I remember lying on the lawn as a carefree child, watching clouds float by and letting my imagination move with them. Thay encouraged us to protect our innocence and made lazy days an essential part of the weekly schedule. These unscheduled days are not indolent; they allow time for personal practice and space for awe and wonder.

Zen is often associated with tea and poetry—the practice of non-practice. In moments of spacious ease, we may notice dead leaves falling, without sadness or regret, dancing on the wind. We may see a barren plum tree fill with spring blossoms. Lazy days, like the sound of a bell, invite us to stop, release our habitual activities, and touch life deeply. This quality of spacious ease can be cultivated in the Eleventh Step.

## The Eleventh Step

> **Step Eleven:** *Sought through prayer and meditation to improve our conscious contact with God as we*

> *understood S/Him, praying only for knowledge of Her will for us and the power to carry that out.*

I grew up as a Jew in name only. I wasn't taught to pray; it wasn't part of my upbringing. But I must have picked it up somewhere along the way because whenever I was in real trouble, I turned to God like an emotional bail bondsman. My prayers were purely transactional. I pleaded and bargained: "Get me out of this!" and offered desperate promises of repentance and better behavior. They say foxhole prayers are the strongest and that hospital walls hear more prayers than churches do. In crisis, the question of who or what God is falls away under the weight of urgency. These prayers come from a raw, unguarded place where intention sharpens and something in us reaches outward.

When I was new to recovery and encouraged to pray, it struck me as religious and made me uncomfortable. But I was willing to try anything that would keep me clean, so I prayed to a god I didn't believe in. My brother's death still rocked me, and praying for him opened the door. I didn't have language for grief or know how to name the ache, but praying for his peace brought me a measure of relief.

At the time, I was sleeping on the couch in Tom D.'s living room, trying to find my footing. Tom had a job and had been clean for a year or two; he was someone I looked up to. One morning, he asked if I had prayed. With a bit of pride, I said, "Yes, I prayed for my brother every day." He looked at me kindly but told me with a bit of steel in his voice, "You should be praying for yourself, Pete. You need all the help you can get."

It was humbling, but I tried. In the mornings, I asked for help staying clean that day. At night, I said thank you. I didn't know who or what I was praying to; if it was just my subconscious, that was enough. In recovery, we're cautioned against selfish or self-seeking prayers, but asking for support to stay clean was appropriate. I heard people talk about their higher power as if they had God in their pocket, even praying for parking spaces. I didn't relate to that, but another saying stuck with me: "Be careful what you pray for, you might get it." The Third Step made it clear: I am not the center of the universe. Trying to manipulate God—or reality—is folly.

The deepest prayers arise from silence rather than words. This is where prayer and meditation meet, where the mind quiets, the heart opens, and presence itself becomes the prayer.

The Eleventh Step has been a bridge from the program into an exploration of Buddhism for many of us. Is Buddhist meditation different from an Eleventh Step practice? Both are paths of understanding and insight. Both cultivate awareness—our conscious contact—which ripens into clarity and a felt sense of wise action, often called God's will.

Do Buddhists pray? That depends on what we mean by prayer. Reciting a mantra, often translated as "mind protection," is practiced in many Buddhist traditions. It's a contemplative refrain that functions much like prayer. A mantra is repeated rhythmically, similar to praying the rosary. Sometimes the mantra is a meaningful phrase; sometimes it is a sacred sound, such as *Om*, an ancient syllable associated with awakening. One of the most widely known mantras is *Om mani padme hum*, the mantra of great compassion in the Tibetan tradition. Through repetition, mantra cultivates wholesome, altruistic states of mind and helps protect the practitioner from afflictive thoughts and emotions such as anger, jealousy, and hatred. Repeating a mantra isn't about asking for something outside ourselves; it aligns the heart and mind.

The male-dominant, Judeo-Christian language of the Eleventh Step was something I had to work through, but the encouragement to improve our conscious contact has always inspired me. It speaks to a latent potential, a capacity for growth that resists complacency. It encourages us to be guided by aspiration and remain on the path, wherever we find ourselves.

The word Buddha means "awakened one." I don't experience God, the Divine, and Buddha as something separate from self. I experience them as our awakened nature—an inseparable aspect of who we are, present within us and all around us as the energy that animates our thoughts, moves the stars, and gives rise to awareness. Awakened nature is our capacity for learning, healing, understanding, and change. It is the light of awareness and love that is always here, always available.

When we cultivate conscious contact with awakened nature, everything has spiritual value. What we experience as obstacles become Dharma doors; what we label poison can become medicine. When met with wisdom, our problems reveal themselves as opportunities to grow, to deepen understanding, and to serve more skillfully.

> *The kingdom of God is available in the here and the now.*
>
> *But the question is whether you are available to the kingdom.*
>
> —THÍCH NHAT HANH

## Mettā Meditation (Loving Kindness)

When I first encountered loving-kindness meditation (Pāli: *mettā*, Sanskrit: *maitrī*), I wasn't sure what to make of it. The traditional phrases sounded like prayer: "May I . . . may she . . . may we . . . may all beings be happy, may all beings be safe." Mettā meditation blurred the line between meditation and something more devotional.

While many forms of meditation focus on attention and concentration, mettā is a heart practice. Its origin story, shared in Buddhist commentaries, is revealing. The Buddha sent a group of monks to meditate in a remote forest during the rainy-season retreat. At first, the forest seemed peaceful, but it was home to tree deities who became unsettled by the monks' presence. The spirits harassed them with foul smells, frightening appearances, and disturbing sounds until the forest felt unsafe. Overwhelmed by fear, the monks returned to the Buddha and asked to be sent somewhere else. Instead of relocating them, the Buddha taught them the Mettā Sutta, the discourse on loving kindness, and instructed them to radiate unconditional goodwill toward all beings, including the very spirits who tormented them. The monks returned to the forest and practiced mettā, offering wishes of safety, happiness, and peace without exception. As the sincerity of their practice deepened, the tree spirits were pacified and later transformed by the warmth and goodwill they encountered. They became protectors of the monks, and the haunted forest became a sanctuary.

There are many forms of loving-kindness meditation practiced across Buddhist and non-Buddhist traditions. What follows is a version adopted by Thich Nhat Hanh, offered with simple guidance:

We begin by directing loving kindness toward ourselves. Until we can care for ourselves with kindness, we have less to offer others. Once that feels steady, we extend the practice outward: to someone we love, someone we like, someone neutral, and finally, to someone who has caused us suffering.

*May I be peaceful, happy, and light in body and spirit.*

*May I be safe and free from injury.*

*May I be free from anger, unwholesome states of mind like fear and worries.*

*May I learn to look at myself with eyes of understanding and love.*

*May I be able to recognize and touch seeds of joy and happiness in myself.*

*May I be able to live fresh, solid, and free.*

*May I be free from attachment and aversion but not fall into indifference.*

## Noble Silence

Noble silence is woven into the life of many Buddhist communities. It's a quiet gift we offer ourselves and one another. We're not forbidden from speaking; we're allowing our internal dialogue to rest. In shared silence, we're freed from the social pressure to fill space with words or respond reflexively. We discover how much can be said with a smile, a gesture, or a nod. Silence becomes a container for deep listening and reflection, a space where we can hear what the chatter of mind and mouth obscures. Our relentless stream of thoughts begins to settle. Noticing the impulse to speak reveals how much of what we say is simply talking to talk: seeking validation, filling pauses, or reassuring ourselves we exist.

In silence, my thirst for connection becomes obvious. When I feel the pull to comment or react, I let it pass. What remains is a quiet presence that doesn't depend on being heard or affirmed. I exist fully without needing to announce myself.

Retreats often include extended periods of silence, sometimes lasting days or weeks. Across traditions, there is a shared understanding: quiet time is spirit time. When the noise fades, something else can be heard: intuition, deeper knowing, the soft voice often buried beneath the debris of busyness.

In the rooms of recovery, we learn the healing power of sharing—breaking isolation through our stories. Noble silence offers a complementary truth: we don't always need to speak to be heard, and we don't always need to be heard to matter. Sometimes the most honest thing we can say is nothing at all.

There is presence in stillness. We hear what we usually miss: the wind in the trees, our own breath, the quiet hum of being alive. Without the ripples of speech, the mind becomes like a calm lake, reflecting clearly. Wordlessness is precious. We touch life directly, with heart-mind, free from the incessant labeling we mistake for reality. When we pass someone on a walking path in silent awareness, something is transmitted that words cannot carry: presence.

Our shared silence deepens concentration. When the mind isn't busy planning what to say, defending, or explaining, attention stabilizes and awareness sharpens. We begin to notice subtle shifts in mood, sensation, and perception usually lost in the noise. This can feel raw at first, even exposed. But it is also freeing. We don't have to be anybody in particular. We are enough—just here, just now.

Noble silence can be a restorative medicine. Many of us in recovery spent years running from ourselves and our pain, often running our mouths along the way. Silence invites us to stop. It is permission to simply be, without performance or pretense. In silence, we touch the peace that was always here. The music of life is revealed, even in our footsteps.

## Walking Meditation

> Solvitur ambulando. *(It is solved by walking.)*
>
> —**ATTRIBUTED TO ST. AUGUSTINE OF HIPPO (354–430 CE)**

I used to think of walking meditation as a secondary practice that was supplemental to sitting. This was a distinction without a difference. Liberation is always and only possible in the present moment, whatever we are doing.

Thich Nhat Hanh introduced walking meditation to the West through the global peace walks he offered as acts of nonviolent resistance to the war in Vietnam. Thay walked in a way that carried a lifetime of practice in every step. I know several people who were so moved by the embodied peace and ease of his footsteps that they went to Plum Village and eventually became monastics.

When I read Thay's talk to inmates, transcribed and published as *Be Free Where You Are*, I knew I had found my teacher. I was enjoying freedom in the program, but Thay's words opened a new door: "Freedom is a practice and a habit. You have to train yourself to walk as a free person, sit as a free person, and eat as a free person."*

We learned to walk by falling, taking tottering steps until confidence grew and we could run. For most adults, walking is a means to an end. We're going somewhere, and our minds are ahead or behind. Walking is something we rarely notice unless we're choosing a parking space or dealing with an injury. Walking mindfully, each step is the destination. We arrive every moment.

In the meditation hall, we practice slow walking, one breath with each step as we circle the sitting cushions. At home, I find a clear space of six to eight feet and walk back and forth, matching my steps to my breath. Breathing in, I feel my foot peeling off the floor and rising; breathing out, I feel it lower, gently caressing the floor as if I were applying a decal. When the mind pulls me away, I pause, return to my breath, and continue. At first, I was rigid with effort, but over time I learned to move with ease.

Sometimes we are too agitated or activated to sit. Walking meditation is grounding and helps me be with strong feelings. In Sister Chân Không's book, *Learning True Love: Practicing Buddhism in a Time of War*,† she repeatedly practices walking meditation when dear friends die and the villages where she built schools and cared for threatened communities were bombed.

Thay showed us that every step is a meditation, whether in our house, on a busy street, or even in the airport. I kept an eye on him when I could, wanting to see if he walked like he talked. One night in India he arrived at our hotel in the middle of the night. I'm not sure what I was doing up and out, but when I saw him, I crept behind him from the lobby to his room, watching. Every step was a poem, even at 2:00 a.m.

---

* Thich Nhat Hanh, *Be Free Where You Are* (Parallax Press, 2002), 16.

† Sister Chân Không, *Learning True Love: Practicing Buddhism in a Time of War* (Parallax Press, 2007).

Outdoor walking meditation is a daily practice in Plum Village communities. Sometimes gathas are used to coordinate breath and steps. Walking outdoors, we take several steps with each in-breath and an equal or greater number with each out-breath. It helps me to silently note "in, in, in" or "out, out, out, out" with each step. This gives the mind something to do while I become present with the sensations of walking and contact with the earth. "I have arrived" (in: arrived, arrived, arrived), "I am home" (out: home, home, home, home) is a favorite gatha. We generally walk a bit slower than usual, but I've covered a lot of ground walking with Thay and the Sangha. Quality of presence does not depend on pace. Joy, ease, and freedom are embodied in our steps. We walk with awareness of those around us, flowing as a river.

I've practiced walking meditation with Thay when more than a thousand of us moved as one body. At times, irritation arose and I struggled. When we're lost in thought, we tend to slow down. That slows everyone behind us. I often notice a tug to speed up, an urgency to "get there" or be at the front. Becoming aware of these movements is the practice.

I remember walking with the Sangha up Vulture Peak (Gṛdhrakūṭa) in Rajgir, India. I was excited to visit the spot where the Buddha delivered several famous teachings, including the Lotus Sutra and the Heart Sutra. The uphill climb was a struggle. I was still sick with liver disease, out of shape, and unaccustomed to the heat and humidity. People—and the occasional cow—moved in both directions as we made our way up the wide stairs and ramps. Surrounded by a sea of brown robes, the color of the Plum Village tradition, I could see Thay about fifty feet ahead. Everyone appeared to move with cool grace while I labored, dripping sweat in my T-shirt and cargo pants.

I wondered what secret monastic training allowed them to glide up the mountain, seemingly without a drop of sweat. In the parlance of AA, I was definitely trudging on the road to happy destiny. My steps grew heavier as I focused on the effort of each step. My attention was stuck on the lifting foot. Stepping over a cow patty, I raised my right foot and noticed my left was at rest. That simple shift eased my way. Pointing my attention to the resting foot rather than the lifting one brought a feeling of freshness. By the time we reached the top, my shirt was drenched, but I was smiling ear to ear.

**Walking Meditation**

*Take my hand.*
*We will walk.*
*We will only walk.*
*We will enjoy our walk*
*without thinking of arriving anywhere.*
*Walk peacefully.*
*Walk happily.*
*Our walk is a peace walk.*
*Our walk is a happiness walk.*
*Then we learn*
*that there is no peace walk;*
*that peace is the walk;*
*that there is no happiness walk;*
*that happiness is the walk.*
*We walk for ourselves.*
*We walk for everyone*
*always hand in hand.*
*Walk and touch peace every moment.*
*Walk and touch happiness every moment.*
*Each step brings a fresh breeze.*
*Each step makes a flower bloom under our feet.*
*Kiss the Earth with your feet.*
*Print on Earth your love and happiness.*
*Earth will be safe*
*when we feel in us enough safety.**

---

* Thich Nhat Hanh, *Call Me by My True Names: The Collected Poems of Thich Nhat Hanh* (Parallax Press, 2022), 236.

## At Ease with Unease

One morning, I was sitting quietly in meditation when my ex-wife came into the adjoining room with my visiting stepdaughter and our baby granddaughter. The little one was wailing, needing her diaper changed. Irritation flared. What's wrong with them? How inconsiderate! Don't they know I'm meditating? The baby's cries were piercing, and my sense of peace evaporated.

Then I thought of Thay sitting in meditation as bombs fell in Vietnam. Breathing in, I calmed myself. What if the baby's cries were simply nature's alarm, signaling that a helpless being needed care? As I sat with the crying, the sound shifted from disturbance to something closer to joy as my meditation steadied enough to hold it. I remembered my visiting stepdaughter was a gift, her infant daughter a treasure. I began to notice the soft, reassuring voices of the adults tending to little Lyla.

As an improvising musician, I know that everything belongs: the bubbling brook, a passing plane, birdsong, soft wind in the trees, and even a wailing infant. Art has always reflected our struggles and shaped something beautiful from suffering. Music is harmony and dissonance, tension and release. The most human way to live is to embrace the full range of experience, remembering that unpleasant moments are just a note in the song. There can be no awakening without slumber.

Getting back into music happened organically. Shortly before my divorce, I started a drug trial, and soon after I was pronounced free of hepatitis C. As my energy returned, I heard the familiar voices of my clarinet and saxophone calling me back. After the divorce, I suddenly had time. I began going out to hear music again and met kindred spirits to play with.

Playing clean and sober felt extraordinary. I had more presence and clarity. Where I once used narcotics to quiet my internal dialogue, mindfulness now helped me harmonize body, mind, and spirit. Music gave voice to my heart where words fell short.

The music, long dormant, was still alive in me, and my fluency returned as I relaxed into the horn again.

Opportunities sprang up without striving. A premier jazz label, No Business Records, contacted me about rereleasing my first album—and even unearthed a recording I didn't know existed. We released an archival set, *No Coming, No Going*, alongside new music from my trio, *The Other Shore*. Both were received with remarkable warmth, and in the years that followed, I recorded several more albums. A dormant part of me had come back to life. To quote from the basic text of Narcotics Anonymous, "Lost dreams awaken, and new possibilities arise."

The return to music was exhilarating and seductive. Part of me yearned to play full-time, but the lure of acclaim fell away. I wanted to keep the music pure—a blessing rather than a vocation. I stayed rooted in what mattered most through my regular commitments with the Prison Meditation Project at Donovan State Prison, local sangha building, the Twelve-Step meeting I brought to the county jail, prison pen-pal work, and my own recovery at the heart of it all.

As life opened up again and I was in the flow, impermanence stopped me cold. On a flight to Seattle for a gig with old friends, I couldn't clear my ears. I was an avid scuba diver, and that had never been an issue. When we landed, I felt weak and sluggish, as if I were underwater. Within a day, my lungs were severely congested. I had a concert in San Diego the next night. I was so sick I could barely stand. I don't know how I got through it—I could barely breathe.

After two days of near-constant sleep, I went to the doctor. They thought it was pneumonia, but I didn't respond to antibiotics. An X-ray led to an emergency CT scan. Two doctors reviewed it on the spot, their expressions setting off alarm bells. When I pressed them to level with me, they said there were lesions across both lungs and my lymph nodes. Based on what they saw, they estimated a 98 percent chance of terminal cancer—and a 2 percent possibility of valley fever, a treatable fungal infection.

It felt like the floor had fallen out from under me. A wave of dread washed over me. My first thought was, "Why me?" A few heartbeats later: "Why not me?" I had sat with the dying. I knew this could come for any of us, at any time. Death is certain; only the time and manner are unknown.

So I did what I knew to do and came back to my breath. Breathing in, I calmed myself; breathing out, I let go. "Okay," I thought, "it looks like this is how I'll go." With surrender, gratitude flooded in—for decades of recovery and a life beyond my dreams. There was a time when I had hoped to die before I got clean; I'd been living on borrowed time ever since. If this was all the life I was to get, it had already been enough. My cup was full.

Weeks later, the results came back: as you may have guessed, it wasn't cancer. After two years of high-dose antifungal treatment, the valley fever infection went into remission, but my airflow and stamina took a serious hit. My music career came to another abrupt halt.

You can't predict how you'll respond to something until you're living it. The stability I felt in the face of a possible cancer diagnosis was the fruit of my practice. Weak from the illness and treatment, I let go of everything: music, prison Dharma work, the county jail meeting, running, scuba diving—so much of what I loved. Who was I now? No longer the prison-Dharma guy or a jazz musician. I was itchy and uncomfortable, shedding a skin, trying to swallow a heaping bowl of acceptance. It felt like loss, but it was also a rebirth, opening doors I couldn't yet see.

How do we prepare for the inevitable? When change comes knocking, it can be shocking, even if we know that flowers inevitably drop their petals. Days turn to night. We live in a world of potential, where every obstacle holds an opening. We can respond as creative improvisers rather than victims, making music out of the noise. Ease is often seen as a reward, but in practice, it is the path, nourishing our capacity to look deeply, again and again. Our limitations do not define us; they invite us to move in new ways.

# PART III

# The Refuge Dwells in Me

We come to the path and learn it before we begin to live it. At first, the changes are dramatic. As our understanding deepens through lived experience, the practices begin to work on us in quieter, more intimate ways. We are the living Dharma, the living program. We are the refuge. We are the song of freedom playing on.

This section moves into deeper waters: the wisdom teachings of the Buddha. I do my best to share them in practical terms. There is nothing to master. This is an uncovering—a lifetime of study and practice for those committed to the path. For those who wish to go deeper, suggested readings at the back of this book offer additional resources.

## THE SIXTH FACTOR OF AWAKENING:

# Concentration

All Buddhist traditions recognize the sixth factor as *samādhi*, which is translated as concentration. But this isn't the kind of concentration I learned in school, squinting at a math problem. Like many ancient terms, the translation only encompasses part of its meaning. Samādhi is also described as unified awareness or meditative absorption.

Thay explained the roots of the word: *sam* means together, *ā* means bringing toward, and *dhi* refers to the energy of the mind. Samādhi is the collected, harmonized energy of the mind.

Recognizing the in-breath and the out-breath is mindfulness. Staying with the entire in-breath or the entire out-breath, without drifting into lunch plans or old regrets, is concentration. Concentration is sustained mindfulness: the mind calmly abiding with its object of attention.

On my first retreat, I experienced moments of deep concentration. When everyone breathes and walks mindfully, the collective energy is incredibly supportive. A retreat offers more than stepping out of routine; we are held by a shared field of practice. Encouraged by my progress, I wondered what distinguishes a Zen master. I realized that while I touch moments of concentration, a master dwells in samādhi more continuously. That encouraged me: every mindful breath adds to the reservoir of concentration.

## Mindfulness, Concentration, and Insight

The words *smṛti*, *samādhi*, and *prajñā* appear in the Plum Village seal and express the living path of practice in this tradition. They are translated as mindfulness, concentration, and insight. Mindfulness brings us home to the present; concentration keeps us there. Concentration is the calm stability of mindfulness, nourished by ease. Prajñā is the insight that develops when the others are present—the fruit of understanding.

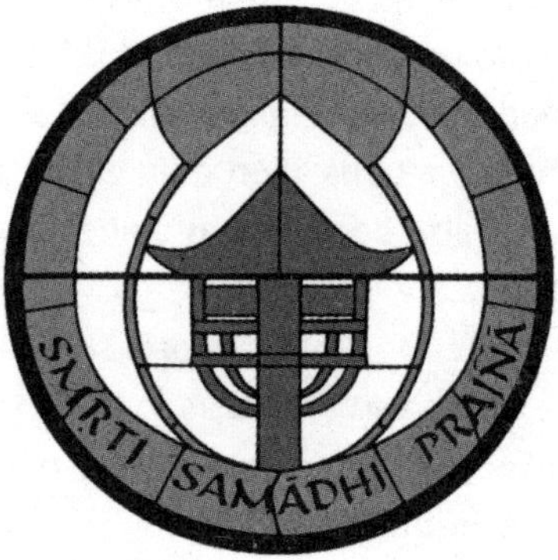


Mindfulness, concentration, and insight inter-are; each contains the others. In concentration, mind and body become one, and we become one with the object of attention. When concentration is strong, we touch the object directly, free of our stories and ideas, discovering its true nature. This clear seeing is insight; when it's fully embodied and guides our actions, it becomes wisdom.

When we begin a sit and turn our attention inward, there is an observer and an observed: "us" and the breath. We are the subject; the breath is the object of our attention. We distinguish the in-breath and out-breath, each with a beginning and an end. As the body calms and the mind settles, attention stays with the whole breath from beginning to end. As concentration deepens, attention no longer rests on the breath—it rests in the breath.

Subject and object, the sense of separateness, fall away. The Buddha described this as mindfulness of the breath in the breath.

A friend once described the program as a submarine. At first, we visit it. Then we climb aboard. Eventually, we live inside it—exactly where we want to be when it's time to go deep as we work the Steps. The Three Refuges feel similar to me. At first, they seem external, something we turn toward. As concentration deepens, we begin to dwell in each refuge. Eventually, we recognize the refuges dwell in us. What once seemed separate is interconnected, and we are no longer trapped by everyday pairs of opposites like self and other. In Buddhist language, this is called the ultimate dimension, where good and bad, in and out, happy and sad are no longer separate entities. They contain one another.

*We are here to awaken from the illusion of our separateness.*

—THÍCH NHAT HANH

If we were truly separate, we could not hear, touch, or communicate with one another. The simple fact that we experience one another reveals the reality of interbeing. The notion of separateness dissolves in experience.

## Right Concentration

Concentration is sustained attention. Our body and mind are unified in the present moment. This can be challenging for those of us who spent years intoxicated and checked out. Concentration itself is neutral; it can serve wholesome or harmful ends. A burglar picking a lock or an addict searching for a vein are both concentrated. The question is what our focus serves.

Right Concentration, the eighth aspect of the Noble Eightfold Path, is concentration directed toward freedom. Guided by mindfulness and wise intention, it leads toward peace, understanding, and genuine happiness. In recovery, Right Concentration reveals the quiet power of surrender, loosening the grip of self-obsession, which the program names as the root of addiction.

In many ways, active addiction is a dissociated state. We disconnect from our bodies, our feelings, our relationships, and our conscience. When we stop using, the pattern of dissociation can persist through phones, social media, shopping, and anything that pulls us away from what is here. Working the Steps, the compulsion to control loosens and the sense of an "I" that manages everything softens. Mindfulness supports a shift from living in our heads to living in our hearts. Are you *at* a meeting, or are you *in* it? Lost in thought, scrolling your phone, taking someone's inventory? Or are you listening with care, feeling kinship and shared humanity? We all know the difference.

The healing power of the program begins with one addict sharing what is truly alive with another: our fears, struggles, experiences, strengths, and hopes. Vulnerable sharing is an antidote to the disease of separation. Deep listening and loving speech belong together. Active listening is more than hearing; it is concentration in action. We attune to tone, rhythm, silence, and gesture with our whole bodies. We hear the music beneath the words. We listen to understand, even when we disagree. This quality of presence—simply here, open, willing to be touched and changed by another—is Right Concentration in everyday clothes. When a person feels genuinely heard, something shifts. Connection is medicine.

Hearts soften when our words are felt rather than simply spoken. When someone says the word "loneliness," we hear. When they feel it as they speak, we are touched. It is a transmission; speaker and listener come together as one. Sadness is palpable; laughter brings laughter. Joy is shared and multiplied.

## May All Be Music

Why is it that we can sit with rapt attention, watching a movie for hours, yet find it hard to settle into a meeting, meditation, or even a conversation? Our absorption in a movie resembles concentration, but it is externally driven and often involves a degree of dissociation. Movies let us escape ourselves. They provide constant sensory stimulation and ask nothing of us. In meetings, meditation, and conversation, we generate our own engagement. When the present moment feels boring or lacking, it is a mindfulness bell. What is lacking is the quality of our attention.

The Seven Factors of Awakening allow us to fully inhabit our lives with breath, presence, and connection. "Present" is a beautiful word. As an adjective it means here and now, and as a noun it means a gift. With mindfulness and concentration, the present is both.

Brother Pháp Hải once shared an Australian children's game called "pass the parcel." A gift is wrapped in layers of paper, with small surprises tucked between them. Everyone sits in a circle, passing the parcel as music plays. When the music stops, the person holding it unwraps a layer and discovers what's there. The game continues until the final gift is revealed. Each moment can be like this, unwrapped with curiosity and joy.

Artists have always tried to wake us up to the ordinary. Andy Warhol did this with his *Campbell's Soup Cans*, and composer John Cage with *4′33″*, a piece in which the pianist opens the lid of the piano, plays no notes for four minutes and thirty-three seconds, and then closes the lid. Listening to *4′33″*, the audience is invited to direct their attention to whatever is present—breath, shifting bodies, creaking chairs—and hear the room itself as music.

Nature makes no distinction between noise and music; we do, shaped by conditioning and inherited ideas of harmony and dissonance, like and dislike, interesting and boring. When we listen without filtering experience, everything can be heard as music. Each moment can be received like a new release from a favorite artist.

Radical presence and radical acceptance give rise to awe. The extraordinary is revealed in the ordinary, the miraculous in the mundane. Freeing ourselves from cultural and habitual bias—decolonizing the mind—means gently releasing learned views that shape our perception. There is no blame; we are developing the awareness to see how history, culture, and habit live in us, and learning to respond freely. Attachment to how we think things should be corrodes our capacity to enjoy things as they are. Mindfulness and concentration open the way to experiencing life directly, with open ears, an open heart, and an open mind. We can sleepwalk through life, bouncing off the walls of our conditioning, or dance to the hidden music with freedom and grace.

**Enter Your Life**

*Enter your life like a great epic poem.*
*Ride the colors of change with the wind,*
*unafraid and unattached.*

*In the light of the coming and going of all things,*
*savor the stars in the dark blue sky.*
*Trust the sun in your heart to guide you home.*

*Here between earth and sky, listen.*
*Hear your own footsteps in the leaves of time.*
*Fix your gaze on the horizon of the not yet, but stay in this moment and ask this great symphony—*
*What is my instrument?*
*What is my music?*
*What is my song?*
*And then surrender to the crucible's alchemy and it becomes the mandala of your holy life.*

*Cross the lake of life's great mystery like a swan*
*embodying grace*
*embodying peace*
*embodying compassion*
*as you head toward the other shore.**

---

* Larry Ward, *Morning Night: Poems on Spirit, Race, and Nature* (Lotus Moss Press, 2025), 55.

## Gathering the Mind

I used to think drugs helped my concentration by quieting my mind while I played music. But narcotizing myself was suppression, not liberation. Addiction fragments the mind; it pulls attention outward and produces dissociated states. Our modern lifestyle does something similar. We're bombarded with information, encouraged to multitask, and our attention becomes scattered. Concentration gathers us back together, restoring the capacity to be wholly present.

It's fascinating that two musicians can use the same instrument and setup, yet each has their own sound. Even pianists, striking identical keys, transmit something distinct. When we are concentrated, our spirit and presence come through the instrument, just as they do through our speaking voice.

Wind players practice long tones, learning to get inside the sound—tuning overtones, developing breath control, and refining tonal quality. I struggled with that discipline and found it boring. I wanted to wiggle my fingers and play a lot of notes. I craved the results but didn't know how to settle and focus. In the early days of my meditation practice, I thought following the breath was boring too. I was focused on the idea of the breath rather than the experience of it. The In/Out, Deep/Slow meditation revealed a shifting landscape of awareness beyond in and out. I had thought of the breath as just a column of air. Now I experience the whole body breathing.

Physical sensations provide a rich field of exploration: the lungs filling and emptying, the ribcage expanding, the coolness of the in-breath and the warmth of the out-breath, the gentle rise and fall of the shoulders, the outward movement of the belly on the inhale and its return toward the spine on the exhale. When I apply mindful breathing to horn playing, the sound comes from my toes.

Counting the breath is a common concentration technique in meditation. At first, I thought the number was what mattered. I chased the goal of five or ten uninterrupted breaths, not realizing the count is only a skillful means to help focus our attention. As my practice developed, I explored other ways of cultivating concentration and arrogantly dismissed counting the breath as something for beginners. I conveniently forgot that I count breaths in walking meditation, tracking how many steps accompany the inhale and exhale. It took me a while to notice that the shift from "in/out" to "deep/slow" is also a form of counting—based on duration rather than numbers. However you arrive at it, you've arrived.

Concentration breathes life into recovery and Buddhist practice. Whether in deep meditation, a conversation, or a meeting, it is the quality of presence that gives each moment its power. Like mindfulness, it grows stronger with consistent practice, deepening our presence in all aspects of life.

There are volumes of teachings on concentration practices in Buddhism. They vary by teacher and tradition and are meant to point the way. They are not things to strive for, attain, or grasp. I'll briefly touch on a few here and invite you to explore more deeply.

## The *Dhyānas*

Long before Siddhartha's awakening, ancient Indian yogis practiced refining concentration into increasingly deeper states of absorption, known as the four *dhyānas* in Sanskrit (*jhanas* in Pāli). Siddhartha studied with two renowned teachers and mastered the four dhyānas, only to discover they did not bring an end to suffering. After his awakening, he taught that these deeper levels of meditative absorption stabilize the mind so liberating insight (*vipassana*)—the key necessity for true freedom—can arise. The dhyānas are a result of deep concentration, not something to strive for.

### The First Dhyāna

Attention rests on the breath or another meditation object, but thinking is still present—you know you're meditating. Perhaps you note the in/out of the breath. You return to your object of concentration as thoughts arise. A sense of well-being may emerge as the mind becomes focused.

## The Second Dhyāna

Discursive thinking ceases and you enter a flow state where attention sustains itself without being directed. Joy deepens, often accompanied by a feeling of freshness and freedom. Sometimes a spontaneous half-smile appears.

## The Third Dhyāna

Joy softens into contentment. You are alert and aware, yet deeply at ease, happy, and unshakable. There is nowhere to go and nothing to do.

## The Fourth Dhyāna

The mind becomes like a still lake, reflecting everything clearly without ripples. Pleasant and unpleasant no longer dominate. What remains is open presence—ideal for deep insight.

These are not exotic states to chase. They arise naturally when the necessary conditions are present and don't always follow in a neat sequence. Like all dharmas, the dhyānas are impermanent. Don't try to force or recapture them. That only creates tension.

## Dhyāna and Recovery

In recovery, progress unfolds through steady engagement. Newcomers often describe "the committee" in their heads—the relentless chatter of racing thoughts. Over time, through meetings, literature, and Step work, the mind begins to settle. The noise quiets. Stability grows. When we begin to feel at home in the program, recovery becomes genuinely alive. Confidence and trust in the path mature. We know who we were, who we are, and who we aspire to be. Having metabolized the Twelve Steps, we're no longer in survival mode. We naturally turn toward helping others and deepening our awakening. Recovery is no longer something we do; it's the way we live. Our life becomes our recovery, and our recovery becomes our life.

When David brought the baby gopher snake home, I figured I'd end up caring for it. I'd kept snakes and lizards as a kid and managed to kill them all. This time, I read up and paid attention.

At the end of long days selling semiconductors, I would stop at the aquarium we'd set up as a cage. Snakes are not very active. My busy mind calmed down as I watched. I was drawn in by the scales, the eyes, the unhurried way the animal moved through its world. I didn't have a name for what I was doing. I now think of it as snake meditation.

Years later, illness ended my job, and my hobby became a livelihood. A career I hadn't planned began with surrender—letting David bring a snake home—and developed by following curiosity rather than a blueprint.

The real teaching came with a species of dwarf monitor lizard from Australia, *Varanus acanthurus*, known as Red Ackies. They looked like animated tribal art—colorful, compact, playful. I was infatuated. But they refused to thrive under the conditions that worked for snakes, and nobody knew why.

We had been providing what we thought they needed, projecting what we knew onto a different animal entirely. Only by watching them carefully—learning to listen without agenda—did the picture change. In their natural habitat, Red Ackies bask in temperatures that would kill a python, but they can also retreat into burrows to regulate their heat. Providing that range, along with the right soil depth for egg laying, was a counterintuitive koan. No amount of research solved it. The answer emerged from sustained, patient attention—from letting go of what I assumed and staying present with what was actually there.

I became the second person in the world to breed this species in captivity. The breakthrough didn't come from thinking harder. It came from thinking less—from dhyāna-like attention: discursive thought ceasing, presence sustaining itself, and something clear arising in the stillness.

The reptile business outlived David. Like all things, it too was impermanent. But it showed me, before I had language for it, what concentration makes possible that intellect alone cannot.

## The Three Dharma Seals: Impermanence, Nonself, and Nirvana

There is no single way to work the Steps. In meetings, I was told the only "must" was not picking up—just for today. Everything else was a suggestion. That gave me room to breathe and eased my fears of dogmatism. Old-timers would add, "If you want what we have, do what we do."

The Buddha offered similar guidance: don't accept any teaching on authority alone—test it in your own life. If something leads to clarity, compassion, and freedom, trust it. Both Buddhism and the Steps are based on direct experience, not blind belief. How the Steps are understood and applied varies from person to person, sponsor to sponsor. As the fellowship spread, Step-working guides emerged to support those without access to experienced members. Some are traditional and published by the fellowships; others offer fresh perspectives, including Buddhist and mindfulness-based approaches. What matters is whether it works in our daily lives.

As Buddhist teachings spread and adapted to local cultures, two main branches emerged. These branches share the same roots but take different approaches to awakening. Theravada carefully preserves the earliest teachings and centers on meditation and personal liberation. Mahayana, which includes Zen and Tibetan traditions, highlights the bodhisattva path of helping all beings awaken. Both offer complete paths to freedom, each with its own flavor.

Twelve-Step fellowships have followed a similar course. The principles are constant, but the language and tone shift to meet the needs of each fellowship. Narcotics Anonymous adapted the language of Alcoholics Anonymous, while Codependents Anonymous shaped it differently. Each fellowship finds its own voice. This is skillful means: crafting a message that truly helps.

It can be confusing when the same teaching appears differently across traditions, but that is part of the Dharma's beauty. One of the qualities I admired in Thich Nhat Hanh was his clarity and depth of understanding. He had a rare ability to express ancient teachings in contemporary language without distorting their meaning or diluting their integrity.

The Three Dharma Seals, foundational insights that reveal the true nature of reality and serve as markers of authentic teaching, are a prime example. You might expect something so essential to be fixed across traditions, but even this varies. In Theravada Buddhism, the Three Dharma Seals are impermanence, nonself, and suffering (*dukkha*). Seeing the instability and unsatisfactoriness of life turns us toward a wiser, kinder way of living. In the Mahayana tradition, the third seal is nirvana instead of suffering. This is not a contradiction but a shift in emphasis. Mahayana teachings highlight that seeing deeply into impermanence and nonself does more than reveal suffering—it points to freedom. Nirvana is not separate from this insight; it is the fruit that ripens from it.

You could say Theravada emphasizes the diagnosis ("this is why we suffer"), while Mahayana points to the cure ("this very understanding is liberation"). Each tradition illuminates the same truths from a different angle.

The Three Dharma Seals are not ideas to believe in or doctrines to defend. They are ways of seeing. We practice concentration on impermanence, nonself, and nirvana, thereby transforming perception and liberating the heart-mind.

## Impermanence

We all "know" about impermanence, but when a shoelace breaks or a tire goes flat, it can still feel unexpected, even personal. There's a world of difference between intellectual understanding and lived experience. We know our friends and loved ones will die, yet we often take them for granted. If we saw with the eyes of impermanence, each person would appear precious and fragile. We would naturally treat one another with more tenderness.

We tend to fear impermanence and resist it. Entire industries thrive on preserving youth and fighting aging. In active addiction, I wanted to feel one feeling all the time. Impermanence was the problem—why do drugs have to wear off? In my ignorance, I craved a stasis that would have denied me the love I've received and the joy of a meaningful life. Impermanence is more than aging, dying, breaking, and wearing out. Thanks to impermanence, life is full of wonders: a seed sprouts, a flower blooms, we get clean, transform suffering, and help others.

In meditation, following the breath is a direct encounter with impermanence. Each inhale and exhale offers the rhythm of birth and death: arising, being, fading, and returning. When the mind is unsettled and attention keeps bouncing off the breath, impermanence can bring peace by reminding us this is just the way it is right now. Otherwise, we freeze a single moment as if it defines the whole movie.

This perspective is foundational to trauma work, which is often part of recovery. Trauma freezes a moment in time and pulls us back into it when we're triggered. Recognizing impermanence, we can metabolize and transform our traumas, fears, and resentments. I've written inventories and forgiven people who caused me harm, only to discover that my forgiveness, too, is impermanent.

I once thought that meant I had failed, but now the resurfacing of resentment may be a gift in disguise—an invitation to practice forgiveness again and come home to my heart. Because of impermanence, awakening is possible—and fleeting. We get to refresh and renew our awakened nature. At times, this can feel like drudgery, but waking up anew is a joy we can learn to delight in, again and again

## Nonself

Nonself is to space what impermanence is to time—it reveals the open, ungraspable nature of what we take to be solid. We spend much of our lives defending and promoting a self that doesn't exist in the way we think it does. We believe we are our thoughts, our feelings, our history, our addiction, our recovery. We introduce ourselves: "I'm an addict," "I'm Pete," or "I'm a Buddhist," as if these labels capture something solid and permanent. But Buddhist teachings on nonself (*anattā*) invite us to look more closely.

In recovery, we discover there is no fixed self, though we may not realize it. The person who drank or used, where did they go? The one who said, "I'll never get clean" or "I can't change," are they still here? We're not the same person we were in active addiction, but we're not completely different either. There's no unchanging self that addiction happened to, only a flowing process of causes and conditions, shaped by everything around us, and inseparable from it.

Nonself doesn't mean we don't exist or that our pain doesn't matter. It means we're not the separate, unchanging "thing" we take ourselves to be. We're more like a river, constantly in motion, made of everything upstream, becoming everything downstream. This is deeply liberating. No matter what we've done or been through, we are worthy of freedom. Our experience can help others. Old shame, resentments, and identities do not define us. They are conditions that change. When someone harms us, we can see they're a person caught in their own stream of causes.

When we relapse, we are not a failed self. We are a process in need of different conditions.

The obsession to use, when examined closely, isn't "mine." It's a visitor, a weather pattern moving through. Cravings arise based on conditions: stress, memory, body chemistry, old neural grooves. When we stop feeding these conditions, they fade. "Our" cravings are more like a song the body-mind plays when certain keys are struck. The Twelve Steps point to this: we admit we're powerless, we become willing, we are transformed through a power not of our own making. Where is the fixed self in that process? Recovery happens through us as we become a channel for healing rather than the hero of our own story.

In meditation, as we contemplate nonself, we inquire: Who is breathing? Who is aware? We look for the one who suffers, the one who recovers, and find only shifting phenomena: sensations, thoughts, feelings, and intentions arising and dissolving in awareness. This can feel unsettling. If there's no solid "me," who is getting sober? But nonself is the root of fearlessness. How can something that was never a fixed entity be destroyed? What can be lost? Seeing our ever-changing nature, we loosen our death grip on "being somebody" and discover the spaciousness of being no particular thing at all—open, responsive, alive.

## Nirvana

In popular culture, nirvana is understood as an untouchably blissful spiritual high—eternal ecstasy and permanent relief from suffering. But in Buddhism nirvana is a cessation: the end of grasping, clinging, and craving. Nirvana isn't the fireworks of a peak experience; it's the peace of surrender, the coolness of abstinence, the stillness of ashes after the fire goes out. In active addiction, we were on fire, burning with desire, consumed by need, inflamed with craving. We chased relief, grasped at pleasure, and ran from pain—and the running itself was the burning.

Nirvana is unconditioned. It is the one thing not dependent on causes and conditions, not subject to arising and passing away. Everything else in our experience is conditioned: feelings respond to thoughts, cravings arise from triggers, moods are colored by circumstances. But the capacity for peace touches something deeper, something not dependent on everything being just right. In recovery, we get a taste of the unconditioned: service that doesn't require recognition, peace that doesn't depend on getting our way, and love that is free from the need to be loved back. When we help another addict simply because our heart responds to their suffering, we touch the unconditioned. There is no expectation, no need for appreciation or credit. When we sit in meditation without grasping or striving, free from the pull of right, wrong, and the drama of self, we touch the unconditioned, cool and clear.

When we turn our will and our lives over in the Third Step, it's not necessarily to an external deity calling the shots, but to this unconditioned nature of love, truth, and reality as it is. We stop trying to bend the world to our fantasies and begin aligning with what's here. The burning stops—not because we finally get what we want, but because we release the wanting. Nirvana doesn't come after enough meetings, steps, or hours on the cushion. It is always here, now, as the breath flows in and out. Awareness itself is untouched by the chaos we mistake for ourselves.

This is the peace, the program and the Dharma promise.

*Just this.*
*Just here.*
*At last, the war is over.*

## Suchness

Toward the end of his life, the Buddha referred to himself as the *Tathagata*—one who has arrived at suchness. Suchness is seeing things as they are, without the filter of craving, fear, or our notions.

It is a deep surrender to truth. Not a passive state but an active peace. Nirvana is suchness.

After my divorce, I practiced coming home to the wholeness of my life just as it was. In recovery, this is called spiritual fitness. When I eventually began dating again, the fire of need, want, and desire easily rekindled. When that happens, we look for a fix. But our true nature is already whole and complete; we don't need someone to complete us. I was happy with my life as it was. What I wanted was someone to share it with. I wanted to enjoy the process rather than grasp for an outcome. I noticed my fantasies and judgments, along with the fear and excitement that felt almost the same in my body. When pangs of despair arose—"there's no one out there for me"—I tried to meet them with love and kindness.

Then I met Betty. On our first date, sparks flew and conversation flowed effortlessly. We shared openly about our lives, God, death, happiness, and sorrow. The first person I dated after the divorce felt like my soulmate. Was it too good to be true? The trauma of divorce brought hesitation, and doubt began to wiggle in my belly. Was I projecting, only seeing what I wanted to see?

The Buddha labeled doubt as a hindrance. Blind doubt is a state of mental paralysis, and with a fear of failure and commitment, I began to fall into it. Thay encouraged to practice with a more helpful reflection: "Am I sure?" This koan invites intelligent investigation—a crucial distinction.

I became sure in the weeks that followed. Betty had ebullient joy, a big heart, and integrity. I had to learn Betty's language of love, to listen deeply with patient spaciousness.

Now it's a life study. We know conflicts are inevitable; we vow to use them as Dharma doors rather than walls. We remind each other that we are here for love; everything else is compost for the garden. And I continue coming home to the wholeness of my life, exactly as it is. This is suchness in action: meeting what is, without the fire of grasping.

## Moments of Wholeness

There are times when I feel that every moment of my life has prepared me for what is called for. Sometimes I know it going into a situation; more often, I understand it only after reflecting on what has transpired. We are the sum total of all our experience, but some moments have added weight and significance.

I worked the first five steps with Hamilton. When I asked him to sponsor me, he smiled and said he would but warned me that no one he had sponsored had stayed clean. I smiled back, relieved that he had said yes, and told him, "I will be the first." Whether it was arrogance or prescience, it turned out to be true. We met in a graveyard for my Fifth Step. He wanted to emphasize the life-and-death nature of addiction and the importance of what we were doing. When I finished, he told me I needed to get a new sponsor because he was moving out of town to live with a woman and open a barber shop. For just a moment, I thought it was personal. Now that he knew my deepest shames and secrets, he was abandoning me. But it was only a fleeting thought. We didn't have cell phones and unlimited calling plans in those days, so I approached Hank Magdaleno, an old-timer who loved jazz. Hank took me through the rest of the steps.

Hank and his wife, Lily, welcomed me into their home, and they treated me like family. I had Sunday dinner with them every week, and Lily made some mean tacos. I had less than a year clean at the time and was still very rough around the edges. I was amazed they wanted me around their three daughters, and being with their family, I gradually started to feel human again. The first Christmas they invited me over for tamales, I was astonished that there was a gift for me under the tree. I wanted to cry but hadn't softened enough for that yet. It was deeply healing to be seen, accepted, and valued.

As part of his amends, Hank had his father living in a converted garage downstairs. I used to call him Grandpa, like the kids did. When he became ill with Parkinson's disease, I watched how Hank and Lily tenderly cared for him. I watched Hank cut his toenails and do other things for him, and thirty years later, I did the same for my father. As Parkinson's progressed, Grandpa was losing functionality, and one day Hank asked if I could watch him for a few hours. I was honored to be trusted and readily agreed. I didn't know what was expected but resolved to do whatever I could. When Grandpa went to the bathroom, he couldn't wipe himself, and I did that for him. It was an act of love that dissolved my limitations.

When Hank died of liver disease, I asked Ham (Hamilton) to sponsor me again. Ham had liver cancer and was waiting for a transplant. I was inspired by his spiritual fitness as he faced the dire powerlessness of his circumstances. His life was held in the balance of circumstances beyond his control, and he remained surrendered, still willing to help others. Twenty-five years later, he was diagnosed with PML, an incurable disease that was destroying the white matter of his brain. Ham had been with me through David's death and supported me through all my major life events. By the time he was ill, I had gone through hospice training and resolved to be with him through his death. It was one of those occasions where I felt that every bit of work and training had prepared me to be there for him. His wife was still working to make ends meet, and I helped Ham eat when he couldn't feed himself, change his clothes, and even wipe himself when he got to that point. It was a rare honor, and I considered it a privilege.

Ham and his wife lived in Arizona, and when I flew home for a weekend to see my wife, I reflected on the prior weeks with Ham and marveled that I could be so unconditionally loving. I wondered if I could ever treat myself with the same kindness, care, acceptance, and patience.

After his death, I went to Deer Park Monastery for a weekend to process and reflect. The Korean sangha had come one night and fed us all. It was great food, a bit spicy, and I must have overeaten. The next morning at the 5:45 a.m. meditation, I was sitting adjacent to the venerable and senior monks when my stomach started to gurgle. I was embarrassed, concerned I might be disturbing them and what they might think of my internal distress. I thought of Ham and the compassion I had shared with him. If it were his stomach, I would meet him with love and concern, bringing comfort rather than shame. It occurred to me that, thinking of Ham, he was alive in my consciousness in that moment, and that if I couldn't love myself that way, I could love the Ham in me as a point of entry. When we care for ourselves, we are caring for all our ancestors and even our descendants.

Years later, I cared for both of my parents in their decline. I cut my father's toenails as Hank had for his father. My brother was astonished and asked how I could even think to do that. I smiled in reply. Thich Nhat Hanh put his lifetime of practice into every word and step. I cared for my parents with all the kindness and tenderness I had ever received.

Someone asked me how long it took to write this manuscript, and my honest reply was seventy-two years. Every moment of our lives is preparing us for the next. Are you wholly ready for this breath and whatever life offers you today?

## The Three Doors of Liberation: Emptiness, Signlessness, and Aimlessness

The Three Doors of Liberation are sometimes called the three concentrations. They are wisdom teachings that speak to the ultimate nature of reality. The words point to something real, but their meaning cannot be grasped through our usual dualistic thinking. Understanding unfolds gradually with study, practice, and deepening concentration.

The Three Dharma Seals are marks of existence that reflect the nature of reality. They are a lens that reveals the Three Doors of Liberation. These doors open into the clarity of Right View, where the flames of greed, hatred, and delusion find no fuel.

Our meditation practice often unfolds along a natural progression: from "I'm learning to sit still and calm my mind", to "I'm seeing the truth of the way things are" (the Three Dharma Seals), to "I'm free" (the Three Doors of Liberation).

When we first encounter the Three Doors, we meet them with the thinking mind—as ideas to contemplate and understand. That's a good beginning. But these teachings are not concepts to collect. They are doors to step through.

The teachings only become real when they move from the head into the body, into our choices, into the way we meet each moment. Understanding begins conceptually, but wisdom flowers through lived experience. The Dharma is a raft: useful for crossing, meant to be released once we reach the other shore. We are not here to accumulate understanding. We are here to be free.

## The Door of Emptiness

In Buddhist teachings, emptiness is not a void, nothingness, or some cosmic vacuum. It means that we are empty of a separate, independent self, that everything is made of nonself elements. Nothing exists without relationship or support. Everything leans on, depends on, and participates in everything else.

This is often termed as dependent origination, or interdependent co-arising. Thay called it interbeing—the fundamental truth that we are inseparable from all that is and that our very presence depends on countless causes and conditions. This insight reveals the Dharma Seals of impermanence and nonself. If nothing exists independently and everything is always changing, there can be no permanent or separate self. Emptiness is the spacious container that holds these truths: the recognition that life arises out of relationships and shifting conditions.

Suffering arises when we mistake a fragment for the whole. We become convinced that a moment of shame proves our unworthiness, or a past action defines our entire identity. We feel alone and cut off—not only from other people, but from our own bodies, our own hearts, and even the present moment. We use substances or behaviors to numb the pain of disconnection.

Touching emptiness is profoundly healing. Our habits, traumas, fears, and cravings are not proof of our unworthiness. They have causes, as the Buddha taught in the Second Noble Truth. Like our joys, hopes, strengths, and resilience, they arise from many conditions. And when conditions change, we change.

Instead of asking, "What's wrong with me?" we begin to wonder, "What conditions gave rise to this suffering?" and "Where did I learn shame?" That shift can be a doorway to freedom.

The nature of interbeing is revealed in all dharmas, including recovery. Everything that arises is a composite, or formation. None of us gets sober alone. We are made of the people who sat with us in meetings, the sponsor who listened at 2:00 a.m., the old-timer whose story cracked our hearts open, the founders and those who came before us, and the friends who show us the way. We are also made of parents, teachers, ancestors, and communities, many of whom we may never meet. We inter-are.

When we see ourselves as empty of a fixed, separate self, we loosen the grip of self-obsession, arrogance, and intolerance. We begin to understand that our healing touches our ancestors and descendants. Our recovery becomes the well-being of the whole fellowship.

When we hold impermanence and nonself within the spaciousness of emptiness, our hearts naturally open to compassion—for ourselves, for our families, and for everyone still suffering. The mind of love is born, and we feel inspired to help others and offer loving service.

## The Door of Signlessness

Signs are the names, labels, and designations we use to make sense of the world—the categories and boxes we place ourselves and others into. We learn signs as we learn to speak. As we do, the brain continuously identifies, catalogs, and interprets sensory input, matching it to what is already known. In Buddhism, this everyday process of naming is called conventional designation.

We get caught in these signs. An unskillful word from childhood can haunt us for decades: lazy, stupid, worthless. Signs can become cages. In the Diamond Sutra, the Buddha stated plainly, "In a place where something can be distinguished by signs . . . there is deception." Thay went further: "Where there is a sign, there is delusion. Where there is perception, there is deception." When we perceive the world, we rely on names, labels, and ideas—but these are only approximations of reality itself.

Signlessness is when we stop mistaking our ideas about reality for reality itself. The sign on the door says "restroom," but the sign isn't the room. The word water will never quench your thirst. Signs aren't wrong; they're incomplete. The sign of a person—their mood, their face, their clothing, their history—is never the fullness of who they are. Signs feel solid, as if they name something absolute. But when we look deeply, we see they are concepts laid over reality—often useful but never the thing itself.

We so easily confuse a sign with reality that it can be challenging to identify our views and notions. The cognitive mind is conditioned to categorize, to pin things down with names. The heart-mind invites us to rest in the direct experience of signlessness, either before naming happens or by recognizing and releasing the label. This includes our experience of feelings. When a feeling arises, we meet it with mindfulness—the feeling in the feeling—free from judgment or interpretation. Without the label, the feeling is less solid, less permanent, less "ours." It becomes weather moving through the sky of the mind.

Thay often taught signlessness through the wisdom of no-birth and no-death. His well-known reminder, "A cloud never dies," points to this truth of continuation. A cloud becomes rain, becomes a river, becomes fog, becomes ice, becomes the moisture in our eyes and the blood in our veins. The cloud transforms but does not die. The signs, not the suchness, change with the form. Looking into signlessness, we see the cloud in our cup of tea rather than thinking the sign "tea" tells the whole story.

We are well practiced in the art of separation. In recovery, we use words like sober, clean, addict, and alcoholic. These can be useful points of identification, but many of us become trapped in them. They are signs that can separate us from one another. Even God and our notions about God are signs, powerful ones. They have caused division and tremendous suffering, both in the rooms of Twelve-Step programs and in the world at large.

The Bodhisattva Manjushri is depicted holding the flaming sword of wisdom. This sword does not divide; it cuts through ignorance, delusion, and duality, revealing our fundamental wholeness and connection. Right Concentration and signlessness are like Manjushri's sword, slicing through fixed views and opening the heart to our original nature: we are the universe, self-aware.

The spiritual principle of anonymity exemplifies signlessness. We welcome all, regardless of age, race, religion, sexuality, or ethnicity. We practice principles before personalities. When we release signs, we truly see one another. Everyone is more than their behavior, more than their wounds, more than their worst day. The newcomer who appears angry or belligerent may be terrified. The old-timer who seems steady may be struggling today. The conditions shaping each moment are vast and ever-changing. Signlessness frees us from the prison of appearances and allows us to meet life as it is: fluid, surprising, and full of possibility.

## The Door of Aimlessness

Aimlessness, the third door of liberation, stops us from running after a better moment, a better version of ourselves, a better life. It frees us from craving, grasping, and the compulsion for specific outcomes, reminding us there is nothing to chase, no permanent result. Aimlessness is the door that opens when we finally stop.

Not because we've given up or stopped caring, but because we realize there is nowhere to be but right here, nothing to become but what we already are. Aimlessness, though, is not passivity or drifting without purpose. It is the razor's edge between aspiration, which arises from wholeness, and desire fueled by a sense of lack.

When we experience the unconditioned nature of the present moment, our deepest needs are met. We are enough. We are released from the burden of expectation and attainment. Everything we have been searching for is already here, in the fabric of the now. This is the soil of aimlessness.

Aimlessness is powerful medicine for our times. Much of our suffering comes from believing happiness lies in the future, something to earn or attain. Addiction is endless running, never arriving, as we chase relief in the next cookie, purchase, high, or distraction. Restless striving can push us to chase serenity as if it were a prize to be won rather than a seed already within us, waiting to be watered. Aimlessness reminds us that freedom is here and now. It is a way of breathing and walking, meeting reality with presence rather than expectation. We are already enough.

Thay distilled this teaching into a calligraphy:

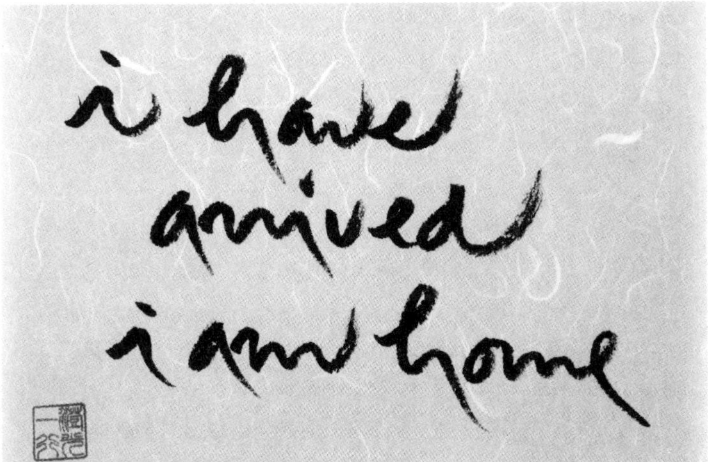

Aimlessness doesn't tell us to abandon responsibility, stop taking action, or dismiss the importance of meetings and service. It invites us to stop living for an imagined future and come home to this moment, where nothing needs to be proven. We act with integrity not to become worthy but because it feels right. We are already worthy—of recovery, of healing, of grace, forgiveness, and love.

Thay offered variations of this theme in his public talks and calligraphies:

> *There is no way to happiness; happiness is the way.*
> *There is no way Home, Home is the way.*
> *There is no way to peace, peace is the way.*

This is the essence of aimlessness. We don't practice to *become* happy—the practice itself is the happiness we seek. We don't get sober so one day life will have value; sobriety is a life of value, right now, right in this challenging, beautiful, ordinary moment.

THE SEVENTH FACTOR OF AWAKENING:

# Equanimity

If mindfulness is the ground of practice, equanimity is the flower that mindfulness blooms. When mindfulness is steady, investigation clear, energy balanced, joy alive, ease present, and concentration strong, the mind ripens into equanimity—a spacious, grounded presence that meets life as it is. Thay initially thought of equanimity as letting go but later came to see it as inclusiveness and nondiscrimination. The Sanskrit word *upekṣā* (Pāli: *upekkhā*) means "to look over" or "to see with a broad view." It is like the perspective from a mountain peak—the vast sky that holds storms and sunshine without attachment or aversion.

Equanimity is not detachment or indifference, nor a transcendent rising above life. It is the capacity to hold everything without clinging to what is pleasant or pushing away what is difficult. It is grounded, engaged, and vitally alive, with warmth and compassion. It is the difference between building walls to protect ourselves and cultivating a heart so spacious it can hold whatever arises without breaking. Rather than "white-knuckling" our way through difficulty, as we say in NA meetings, we meet each moment with curiosity and interest, as a Dharma door.

Indifference is a "near enemy" of equanimity. They may look similar on the surface, but indifference is emotionally flat and disconnected. True equanimity is engaged and present. It is not passivity in the face of injustice; it provides stable ground from which wise, skillful action arises. From equanimity, we speak out, show up, and take action with love and clarity rather than anger and intolerance.

The Buddha taught four kinds of equanimity, each essential in recovery to help us meet cravings, aversions, emotional surges, and the unpredictability of life with balance and clarity:

1. Equanimity amid the Eight Worldly Winds: gain and loss, praise and blame, pleasure and pain, fame and disrepute.
2. Equanimity toward all beings: not elevating some or rejecting others.
3. Equanimity in meditation: a calm, collected presence that sees the impermanence of all things.
4. Equanimity of wisdom: seeing things as they truly are, beyond fixed ideas and illusions.

Equanimity is the deep steadiness that allows us to ride the waves of life without capsizing. It is an underlying principle of the Twelfth Step: we carry the message to all who suffer, without discrimination. We hold their joys and heartaches without losing ourselves. We practice spiritual principles inclusively, in all our affairs, aligned with our highest aspiration.

Our spiritual fitness has limits; it depends on our resilience. We find balance within the zone of recovery.

## The Zone of Recovery

The Buddha once gave a teaching on the bank of a river. He held up a cup of salt and a cup of water. "If I pour this salt into the water," he asked, "will it be safe to drink?"

A student replied, "No, it would make you sick."

The Buddha nodded. Then he gestured toward the river flowing beside them. "If I pour the same salt into this river, would the water be safe to drink?"

"Yes," came the answer. "The river is vast."

This teaching underscores an essential point: the size of our container matters. When my mind is open and my heart is spacious, the small stuff doesn't get under my skin. Quirks, delays, and random annoyances—even other people's flaws—become tolerable, sometimes even endearing. But when I'm tight and constricted, when my heart is the size of a teacup, even a grain of salt can feel like poison.

In recovery, we describe the difference between the teacup and the river as our "spiritual fitness." Practices like mindfulness, ease, joy, and concentration—what the Buddha called the Factors of Awakening—support this fitness. They nourish our peace and stability, even the state of nonfear known as nirvana. But our spiritual condition is impermanent and requires daily attention. What bumps us out? Part of the answer lies in understanding our nervous system—the layer beneath our thoughts and emotions that quietly shapes our experience.

Our senses supply a constant stream of information, whether we're aware of it or not. Operating largely outside conscious control, our autonomic nervous system filters this stream, scanning the environment and our internal state for signs of safety or danger. When we feel safe—in our "window of tolerance" or "recovery zone"—our parasympathetic nervous system engages and the body can rest, digest, heal, and connect. Our heart rate settles and our breathing deepens. We can think clearly and feel curiosity, openness, and compassion for ourselves and others. This is the neurobiological ground from which spiritual fitness can stabilize and grow.

But when the system detects a threat, whether real or imagined, everything changes. The sympathetic nervous system activates and we enter survival mode. Adrenaline is released. Heart rate and blood pressure spike. Blood diverts from digestion to large muscle groups, preparing us to fight or flee. Our ability to connect diminishes. Thinking becomes rigid and reactive. The prefrontal cortex—the part of the brain that allows for mindfulness, perspective, and wise response—goes offline. The riverbed dries up, and suddenly we're a teacup: bracing, flinching, snapping, shutting down. In this state, equanimity isn't just difficult—it's neurobiologically unavailable.

In addition to a fight-or-flight response, our system can shift into a kind of shutdown when we sense an overwhelming threat and escape seems impossible. In this freeze state, heart rate and blood pressure drop. We feel numb, dissociated, and helpless. Endorphins rise to help us endure, but we lose access to facial expression, eye contact, and social connection.

Most of us are intimately familiar with these states. We've spent years oscillating between the hypervigilance of a fight-or-flight response and the numbing shutdown of a freeze. We may have even mistaken that frozen state for serenity, confusing dissociation with the peace we sought through drugs, meditation, or spiritual practice.

There are subtle ways we feed fear and allow it to suppress the goodness of connection, expression, and vulnerability. When we want to share in a meeting or Dharma circle and don't, what is blocking us? It's a form of freeze. We haven't gone offline, but we've empowered the fear and let it immobilize us.

There is another, more subtle behavioral expression of fear known as fawning. It can feel like safety, but it is far removed from authentic connection. Some people call it people-pleasing. I used it as a form of manipulation, but it is also a placating behavior we slip into when we feel unsafe. We may even use an internal form of fawning to soothe ourselves, putting a smiley face on things or covering uncomfortable feelings with spiritual platitudes. This is known as spiritual bypassing, a real danger. It is sometimes linked to what is called "spiritual arrogance." While conditions for joy and safety are often available, we turn toward them to nourish resilience and support our capacity to be present with suffering—not to avoid it.

Practicing mettā meditation, I have bypassed my discomfort by sending loving kindness "at" someone when I wasn't feeling it. Buddhism teaches us to practice loving kindness for ourselves before extending it to others, first offering it to the parts of ourselves that are angry, hurt, or upset. We need to restore our well-being to authentically share the loving medicine of our hearts with others.

Understanding the physiology of the nervous system brings liberating awareness. I remember going on a long retreat and feeling deeply grounded in my practice. I felt a deep sense of community, and my heart was full of love and gratitude. Driving home from the monastery, someone cut me off or wouldn't let me change lanes. In a heartbeat, I was cursing them and making crude hand gestures—without a conscious thought. It hadn't been more than fifteen minutes since I left the retreat, and my serenity was gone. The anger turned inward and self-recrimination followed. I thought my practice was a sham, and I was filled with shame.

Understanding that my reaction was an autonomic response of the nervous system came as a relief. The nervous system is not an enemy; its fear responses are its language of love—sometimes an ignorant love but one that seeks to protect us and ensure our safety nonetheless.

When we find ourselves anxious, agitated, or shut down, we're not failing. Our nervous system is simply doing what nervous systems do when they perceive threat. We can smile to comfort our nervous system. We have the capacity to harmonize it, to calm and care for it. The Buddha used the example of a lute string. When the string is wound too tightly, the instrument is out of tune—the notes are abrasive and disturbing. When the string is too loose, its sound is dull and listless. When the strings are properly tuned, each note is resonant, full of harmonious overtones; it rings and sings.

When the nervous system is in harmony, we resonate with goodness, and a fifth "f state" called flow can arise. Artists of all kinds know this as a state of vibrant creativity, with focus and ease. In flow, we use all the ingredients of our lives with equanimity to express our spirit. We may feel like a channel for the ancestral stream or the divine, connected to the greater self.

We can't turn equanimity on with a button, but we can cultivate the conditions that allow it to arise. It is helpful to recognize our neurological state and notice when we need a harmonic adjustment.

The largest neurological "string" we can tune on our lute is the vagus nerve, which connects the brain to the heart, lungs, and digestive tract. It plays a crucial role in regulating many of the body's automatic functions. It sends signals of safety and calm that influence heart rate, breathing, mood, and stress. When the nervous system is activated by fear or threat, the part of the brain that supports mindfulness and wise response can go quiet.

Practices like deep breathing, walking meditation, or gentle rocking can help calm the nervous system. We are actively shifting our neurobiological state, creating the conditions for mindfulness and equanimity to emerge. A regulated nervous system is what some call the zone of mindfulness.

Humming is a particularly effective way to calm the nervous system and quiet the mind. When I am unsettled as I approach the meditation cushion, I often begin with a minute of humming. When we have a tough decision to make, we may naturally pause with a "hmmm." When my wife and I are at odds, we often pause to hum for a minute or two. It helps us let go of resistance and regain some spaciousness. It's a great practice any time: musical, harmonious, oxygenating, and uplifting.

Since the nervous system is invisible, I look for clues that point me to it. Am I reacting or responding? Is my attention on loving or on who isn't loving me? A spot-check like this reminds me that I am not a victim. I can recalibrate at any time.

Our capacity to help others depends on our own condition. As the Buddha put it,

*If one going down into a river,*
*swollen and swiftly flowing,*
*is carried away by the current,*
*how can one help others across?*

—SUTTA NIPATA 2.321

We don't need to pathologize our experience or reduce spiritual practice to neuroscience. But this understanding can help us remember that we are whole beings, body and mind inseparable. A settled nervous system supports a settled mind. From that settling, the vast heart of equanimity can naturally unfold.

## The Brahmavihārās

The *brahmavihārās*, or "divine abodes," are loving kindness, compassion, sympathetic joy, and equanimity. They are also known as the four immeasurable minds, because when fully developed, they know no bounds—they ripple outward without limit. Thich Nhat Hanh referred to them as the four qualities of true love:

- *mettā* (Sanskrit: *maitrī*, Pāli: mettā)—loving kindness
- *karuṇā* (Pāli/Sanskrit)—compassion
- *muditā* (Pāli/Sanskrit)—sympathetic joy
- *upekṣā* (Sanskrit: *upekṣā*, Pāli: *upekkhā*)—equanimity

They are both a practice and a fruit of practice. The Buddha presented them as spiritual medicine, each one functioning as an antidote to an unwholesome state, sometimes called the four unwholesome abodes:

| Quality of the Heart | Counteracts |
|---|---|
| Loving Kindness | Hatred/Ill Will |
| Compassion | Cruelty /Indifference |
| Sympathetic Joy | Envy/Jealousy |
| Equanimity | Craving/Aversion |

## Loving Kindness

Loving kindness is the sincere wish that all beings, including ourselves, be happy, free from affliction, and at ease. When Stephen Levine first introduced me to mettā practice, I didn't believe I was worthy, but his soulful language inspired and softened my inner resistance. For me, mettā and self-compassion were graduate-level recovery work. I was entrenched in the wrong view of separateness and shame. Then he pointed out that if an injured bird, animal, or crying infant is worthy of care, so are you—and so am I. My heart opened. We don't have to qualify for loving kindness.

## Compassion

Karuṇa, the second element of true love, is the capacity to be present with suffering and the heartfelt intention to help ease it. It arises naturally when we touch our own deepest nature. If you close a door on your finger, your other hand will immediately reach for the injured finger, holding it tenderly to offer comfort and ease the pain. There is no fear of reprisal or need for apology—just an instinct to care. This is compassion, which is different from empathy. Empathy *feels with*: we understand and share another person's feelings. Compassion *responds* to lessen or remove suffering and offer healing. Thay taught that compassion is like a protective armor that allows us to be with suffering, ours or others,' without becoming overwhelmed.

## Sympathetic Joy

Muditā, the third element of true love, is the joy we feel for others. It's the gladness that arises when we witness someone else's success, healing, or happiness. Instead of contracting and feeling diminished by another's good fortune, we expand and feel genuinely delighted for them. When we are spiritually fit—living from abundance rather than lack—there is plenty to go around. Mudita differs from pīti, the fourth factor of awakening, only in its cause: the former is caused by another's well-being; the latter, by a state of deep concentration. The experience of joy, however, is the same.

There are sweet moments in recovery: when we see a newcomer "get it," and the light goes on in their eyes, our hearts naturally fill with joy. When someone who has struggled—or someone we sponsor—celebrates a year clean, when someone reconciles with a family member, regains custody of a child, or when anyone in the fellowship finds freedom, their victory becomes our joy. There is no scoreboard. No "why them and not me?" Sympathetic joy is a pure appreciation for the blooming of freedom wherever it appears.

## Equanimity

These four qualities nourish one another. Equanimity keeps the heart open to all. It is the quality of nondiscrimination, of radical inclusiveness. It allows us to love not only those we find easy to love—babies, puppies, and friends—but also the difficult ones: the stranger, the betrayer, those who have caused us harm. It is the strength that lets us stay present with tender care for a loved one's suffering without fixing or fleeing, even when we're exhausted or the suffering feels endless.

With equanimity, the field of loving kindness extends from self-love to those close to us and outward to all beings: the living and the dead, the two-legged, the four-legged, and the legless, those who fly and swim, the born and the not-yet-born.

Equanimity is the spaciousness that allows the other three qualities of true love to become immeasurable. When the first three brahmavihārās are embodied, the equanimous heart naturally opens, like the vast sky that holds a cloud. When equanimity touches these other qualities, they become vast loving kindness, vast compassion, and vast sympathetic joy (*mahā-maitrī, mahā-karuṇā, and mahā-muditā*).

## True Love

Love is not something we have to manufacture. It is what remains when we stop contracting in fear. When the nervous system rests, the heart opens. As our awakening deepens, so does our capacity for love. First, we begin to accept ourselves just as we are. Then, often to our surprise, we begin to like ourselves. Living with integrity and working the Steps, we learn to care for ourselves. In time, we come to love ourselves—often the hardest love after years of shame and self-recrimination—and that love begins to ripple outward: to our recovery community, to those who "get it" and to those who relapse; to family members who didn't understand; to the people who harmed us; to strangers on the street; to all beings who suffer and long to be free.

The heart's capacity to grow is without limit. There is always room for more salt in the river.

> *The Buddha said that the Four Immeasurable Minds of love practiced with the Seven Factors of Awakening bring Complete, Perfect Enlightenment. The Seven Factors of Awakening are, therefore, the practice of love.**

# Not Knowing, Bearing Witness, and Loving Action

Before finding a home in the Plum Village tradition, I practiced Soto Zen at the Sweetwater Zen Center, where I encountered the

* Thich Nhat Hanh, *The Heart of the Buddha's Teaching* (Parallax Press, 1998), 202.

Zen Peacemaker lineage and its three tenets: not knowing, bearing witness, and loving action.

These tenets are living principles—an invitation to meet life with presence, humility, and integrity. Together, they form both a path and an expression of equanimity in action. When we lose our way, they become guideposts that point the way home.

## Not Knowing

Not knowing is the willingness to meet each moment, each person, each situation with fresh eyes rather than through filters of assumption or judgment. With the spaciousness of beginner's mind, we meet the "great mystery" with peace instead of fear. Thay said, "Knowledge is the greatest obstacle to awakening." When we cling to what we know, we limit fresh insight. Asking "Am I sure?" softens our grip on even our most cherished certainties—the stories we tell ourselves about how things are or how they ought to be.

In recovery meetings, not knowing softens our judgments. When someone shares the same struggle week after week, seemingly stuck or unable to try a solution, we may think they're not really working the program. But applying the principle of not knowing, we ask: "What don't I yet see? Their path isn't mine to walk. Can I release my assumptions about what healing should look like for them?"

Ram Dass said, "If you think you are enlightened, go spend a week with your family." In family dynamics, not knowing can be revolutionary. Do you ever enter a conversation convinced you know what someone will say? Or find yourself rehearsing a defense in anticipation of an attack? It's easy to do with family because we "know" them so well and draw on a lifetime of history. But haven't there been moments when we felt heard and understood? Not knowing invites openness, spontaneity, and curiosity.

## Bearing Witness

From the open ground of not knowing, we bear witness to things as they are, without our mental constructs. This is wholehearted presence, not quiet indifference or passive observation. We listen with our entire being, attentive to what is seen and heard, to what is spoken and what is left unsaid, to tone, silence, body language, and everything in between.

When we bear witness to individual, systemic, personal, and planetary suffering, we don't turn away or drown in it. We sit with injustice without hardening into rage or collapsing into despair. We listen to a loved one's pain without rushing in to fix it. This spacious presence becomes a healing connection, allowing us to see what is truly needed rather than react from anxiety.

When we bear witness with the vast, nondiscriminating heart of equanimity, we can stay present with the difficult person, the tiresome complaint, or the overwhelming tragedy without losing ourselves. We remain grounded. We keep listening.

## Loving Action

Loving action arises from not knowing and bearing witness—not as an impulse, fix-it strategy, or bid for merit, but as the natural outflow of an equanimous heart. Action born of equanimity is wise and discerning. The right medicine may be a kind word, silence, a hand on someone's shoulder, or a step back.

There is a delicate line between helping and enabling, compassion and codependence. Equanimity allows us to see that line clearly and navigate it with care. Sometimes loving action takes the form of fierce compassion and may involve setting boundaries or saying no.

We see this symbolized in the two guardian figures outside many Eastern temples: one peaceful and serene, the other fierce and wrathful. Both are expressions of love. The peaceful bodhisattva offers refuge; the fierce protector stands their ground.

## A Way Home

In December 1985, I was standing at a pay phone in Santa Monica, trying to sell stolen recording equipment, when I heard the news that my brother Richard had shot himself. When it happened, I had been locked up. I went numb from the news; it felt as if the ground had fallen out from beneath me. Late afternoon had turned to dusk, and a chill was creeping into the air—and into my bones.

My family had cut off all contact with me, but now, I thought it would surely reopen. I called my parents, looking for refuge, and they calmly told me the details. This was the first time we had spoken in a year, and it was good to hear their voices. I mumbled something and told them I would be right over. They had lost one son—how could they refuse another? But my mom said, "You are not welcome here. Call us when you've been clean for a year." This clear boundary hurt. And it helped. I got clean a few weeks later—their tough love saved my life.

Not knowing, bearing witness, and loving action remind us that spiritual practice isn't about rising above life—it's about showing up fully for it. With a steady heart, we stay open even when things get hard. Because equanimity is impermanent, it can seem to disappear when we're triggered or contract from judgment and fear. The three tenets offer us a way home. When we notice we've lost our balance, we return to not knowing. We can practice bearing witness again. And from that ground, loving action shows the way forward—again and again.

The three tenets inform my Third-Step koan: "What does love look like here?" That question comes to life in Step Twelve.

# Love in Action

> **Step Twelve:** *Having had a spiritual awakening as a result of these steps, we tried to carry this message to addicts, and to practice these principles in all our affairs.*

It's bold to claim that working the Steps will result in a spiritual awakening. The founders were sure of themselves. When I first read the step, I imagined superpowers or cosmic consciousness—a permanent, exalted state of perfection. Later, when I arrived at Step Twelve, still flawed and struggling, it felt anticlimactic. Disappointed and vaguely ashamed, I dismissed the phrase "spiritual awakening" and focused instead on the second half of the step: carrying the message.

That part I understood. I knew how to show up for other addicts, how to share experience, strength, and hope. Offering the gift of recovery felt noble, useful, and empowering. I had arrived destitute, but now I had something of value to share.

I became obsessed with sponsoring other men and being of service. Once a self-obsessed addict, I now genuinely cared about newcomers and the welfare of the fellowship. Helping others gave meaning to my life. I felt worthy and validated. Even so, stuck in preconceptions of an exalted state and unable to see my own transformation, I kept pushing away the notion of "spiritual awakening." Once again, I concluded I was too broken to experience goodness. I didn't realize that loving service is the natural expression of spiritual awakening.

Meditation practice helped me look with fresh eyes. I saw that the step's wording had derailed me. "Having had" sounded like something finished. I read it as an arrival or final destination. But spiritual awakening, I came to see, is a verb, not a noun. It is an unconstrained movement of the heart, an opening of spirit that unfolds and develops. A spiritual awakening doesn't make us more than human. It makes us fully, vulnerably, and beautifully human. When we bump up against our limitations, we resolve to learn from them. Mistakes become trail markers, revealing where we can deepen our understanding or grow more skillful.

If there is something we call spiritual awakening, there must also be spiritual slumber. They are two sides of one coin. Our forgetfulness is not cause for shame or proof of unworthiness. It's simply the truth of impermanence.

In Twelve-Step parlance, we carry the message of recovery to other addicts and alcoholics. But what is the message? It begins with freedom from active addiction and blossoms into something even more profound: an ineffable awakening of spirit, transmitted through presence, freedom, steadiness, and care.

The last part of the Twelfth Step reminds us to practice these principles in all our affairs. What we learn in Twelve-Step meetings, we bring into the world. Everything has spiritual value. I felt so flawed, often impatient and unkind, that trying to live up to these principles felt like a recipe for failure. So I didn't try. Ironically, my fear fed the shame I was trying to avoid.

The Twelfth Step is an aspirational heart practice. Our aspiration is unconditioned; it is not touched by causes and conditions, does not demand perfection, and is not tarnished by our imperfections. We are called to embody boundless love without discrimination. "Practice" is the operative word—in recovery and the Dharma.

We will fall short and cause harm through ignorance, unskillfulness, or forgetfulness. These missteps can refine rather than define us; they can deepen our clarity and strengthen our resolve. We cultivate this aspiration and let it animate our being. There is no failure.

The heart's deepest desire—to align our whole being with what is most noble—is itself an exalted state, a moment of nirvana, free of outcome, boundless.

The Steps point us toward moments of total surrender—moments when the heart writes a check that can never be cashed, and we commit fully. These are moments of embodied aspiration, distinct from results.

We find them in the decision and surrender of Step Three, becoming entirely ready in Step Six, the humility of Step Seven, the willingness of Step Eight, the courage of Step Nine, the deep listening and surrender of Step Eleven, and the aspiration and transmission of Step Twelve.

I've learned to recognize the moments I align with this aspiration as sacred—I pause to feel them fully and imprint them in my body as a living resource. Just as I remember hitting bottom in my bones, I anchor the felt sense of grace and clarity so I can return to it. Moments of embodied aspiration become the setting for my spiritual GPS. When I drift off course, I recalibrate, finding my way home again and again.

## The Great Vow

Working the Twelfth Step, we step onto the bodhisattva path. A bodhisattva lives in the world, engaged in concrete actions to help all beings—an awakened one who embodies and continually develops the Six Perfections (generosity, ethical conduct, patience, diligence, concentration, and wisdom). Bodhisattvas are not distant deities; they represent archetypal energies and awakened qualities we already possess and aspire to cultivate more fully. I call upon these qualities for support, guidance, and refuge.

In many Buddhist traditions bodhisattvas appear in statues and scrolls, not as objects of worship but as sources of inspiration that remind us the seeds of awakening are within us, waiting to bloom. In Mahayana Buddhism, the most widely honored bodhisattvas go by different names in different cultures and languages but express the same qualities of awakening:

Manjushri—Bodhisattva of Great Wisdom, wielding the flaming sword that cuts through ignorance and delusion. Manjusri's wisdom is not cold intellect, but clear seeing that liberates.

Samantabhadra—Bodhisattva of Great Action, symbolizing the vow to work mindfully, joyfully, and tirelessly for the benefit of all beings.

Avalokiteshvara (Kannon, Kanzeon, Guan Yin, Chenrezig)—Bodhisattva of Great Compassion and Deep Listening, often depicted with a thousand arms or eyes representing compassion paired with the insight to respond skillfully in every direction.

Kshitigarbha (Jizō)—Bodhisattva of Great Vow (Aspiration), fearless and persevering, entering the deepest realms of suffering and vowing not to rest until all beings are free.

Maitreya—Bodhisattva of Loving kindness, the Buddha-to-be, often depicted as the laughing, rotund figure embodying patience, generosity, and joyful abundance—loving kindness available now.

Sadaparibhuta, the Never-Disparaging Bodhisattva, bows to everyone, saying: "I do not dare to underestimate you, because I see you will become a Buddha." Inviting us to look beyond behavior and see the light within.

In the Plum Village tradition, we recognize the Earth and Sun as bodhisattvas:

Gaia, Mother Earth—embodying patience, solidity, nonjudgment, and unconditional love, offering herself freely without discrimination.

The Sun—offering light and warmth to all beings without needing recognition.

There are countless bodhisattvas named in the sutras. We are all bodhisattvas in training. They aren't confined to sacred texts; they show up in ordinary, imperfect, human ways. Zen teacher Joan Sutherland invites us to notice our own everyday bodhisattvas: Fingers-Crossed Bodhisattva, Pretty-Close Bodhisattva, Not-a-Bad-Morning Bodhisattva, Flying-by-the-Seat-of-My-Pants Bodhisattva.

In recovery, we know these energies intimately. A few we might meet:

- The Bodhisattva of Showing Up
- The Bodhisattva of Setting Up the Meeting
- The Bodhisattva of Putting Away Chairs

- The Bodhisattva Who Always Welcomes Newcomers
- The Bodhisattva of Giving Rides to Meetings
- The Bodhisattva of Making Coffee
- The Bodhisattva of Carrying the 1Message

As Brother Pháp Hải reminds us: "A bodhisattva is someone who befriends all things—even, or perhaps especially, the people, experiences, and parts of ourselves we're afraid of." A bodhisattva vow expresses a spiritual ideal and a great aspiration. There are many versions of the Four Great Vows. Here is Thich Nhat Hanh's rendering:

> *The awakened way is unsurpassable; I vow to embody it.*
>
> *However innumerable beings are, I vow to meet them with kindness and interest.*
>
> *However inexhaustible the states of suffering are, I vow to touch them with patience and love.*
>
> *However immeasurable the Dharmas are, I vow to explore them deeply.*
>
> *However incomparable the mystery of interbeing, I vow to surrender to it freely.**

These vows are impossible to complete—and that is their power. We're not promising success. We're orienting our whole being toward an infinite horizon. The impossibility doesn't diminish the vow. It sanctifies it.

The Twelfth Step is a program version of the Bodhisattva Vow. It invites us to commit to the unattainable: to help the addict in distress and to practice spiritual principles in all our affairs—whether in the meeting rooms, the car, or the bathroom. The bodhisattva vow and the Twelfth Step transform ordinary life into a sacred practice.

---

* Thich Nhat Hanh, "The Vows of the Four Great Bodhisattvas," Dharma Talk given at New Hamlet, Plum Village, January 15, 1998.

As I was typing this, the phone rang. I was focused, riding the flow of writing. My nervous system registered the sound as an interruption, but I saw it was someone I sponsor. "I" didn't answer the call—the Bodhisattva of Sponsorship did. The call wasn't urgent, so I bowed off with care. Then the Bodhisattva of Renewed Concentration gently returned me to the page. And now, the Bodhisattva of Always Having More to Say meets the Bodhisattva of Wise Discernment, and this section comes to a close with a blessing: may we continue to clarify the jewel of our aspiration, take refuge in it, and walk the Bodhisattva Path with equanimity and joy.

## Shining Light: A Practice of Equanimity and Love

Thay suggested that the next Buddha, Maitreya, might manifest as the Sangha, rather than an individual. We need a loving community to stay steadfast on the path. Plum Village has a practice called Shining the Light, in which the community illuminates both our strengths and areas we can grow. In recovery, a sponsor often offers similar reflection. As a Sangha practice, Shining the Light draws on "sangha eyes," the collective wisdom of the community, which sees more clearly than any one of us alone.

Shining Light is not a "calling out," but a calling forth that requires deep listening, loving speech, and equanimity. If we hold a grudge or have a bone to pick, we are encouraged to request a Beginning Anew ceremony instead and refrain from speaking during Shining Light. We shine light so the recipient can realize the highest fruits of the practice.

Monastics traditionally engage in this practice at the end of the annual three-month Rains Retreat. In the lay community, Shining Light is often offered before an aspirant receives ordination. Each sharing begins and ends with flower watering—naming the qualities we admire and appreciate in the person. Then, if appropriate, we offer reflections on what may be blocking their joy: unwholesome habit energies or blind spots that can cause suffering. The ratio of flowers to growing opportunities is usually four or five to one. Those offering guidance speak with humility, aware their perception is limited. We remember that we, too, may have contributed to the other person's difficulty. We shine light not as outsiders, but as participants in the interwoven web of practice and relationship.

The recipient listens deeply in silence. This is a time to receive, not to respond. Equanimity allows us to receive everything shared—praise, discomfort, confusion, gratitude. Even if we disagree, we listen carefully and reflect deeply, taking time to consider and bow to the offering.

Shining Light is deeply healing. It builds unity, strengthens trust, deepens insight, and reminds us that we are all here to grow together. It invites a broad perspective that embraces joy and sorrow, success and struggle, light and shadow. We hold ourselves and one another, not shrinking from what is hard to see, but expanding enough to see it with love. As Thay wrote, "When we look after the other person, we are looking after ourselves."

## Unconditional Love

I suffer in the aftermath of an election. The relentless news cycle pushes fear like a chaotic symphony: drums of intolerance, trumpets of grandiosity, cymbals crashing with outrage. Beneath it all, I strain to hear the subtler voices: strings carrying the grief of the marginalized, muted tones of the oppressed, and bass lines holding a steady pulse of resilience. It's a cacophony—and somehow, also a prayer.

I ride the waves of outrage and sorrow—sometimes pulled under by the salty undertow, sometimes rising on the raft of mindfulness and impermanence. Breathing in, I smile. Breathing out, I smile. Powerless. Unmanageable.

What does love look like here?

How do I return to meetings and stay present with people who voted for values that seem to threaten inclusivity, non-harming, compassion, and care—core values of our fellowship, where love and tolerance are our code?

Listening deeply, I notice the cricket's song hasn't changed. The birds still sing. The wind in the trees continues its timeless music. My dog's tail thumps against my chair in quiet contentment. The scent of roses and herbs lingers in the morning light. The sun rises and shines on everything—quietly, faithfully.

Empires rise and fall, but the earth remains steady beneath our feet, allowing me to touch something enduring. She doesn't dismiss the suffering of the world but holds it in a wider field of awareness. In that space, the layers of fear that have taken root in me become clear. Fear for the sick, vulnerable, and marginalized; for the poor and the unhoused; for communities of color; for queer and transgender people; for the arts, Earth herself, and all sentient beings. My deep care, strained under the weight of discrimination and polarization, has curdled into an afflicted state of anxious overwhelm. How can I bring compassion and balance to this inner storm? How do I hold this with tenderness rather than tension?

Breathing mindfully, my concentration deepens. Mind and heart become one. Thoughts of right and wrong, like and dislike, fall away. I come home to the heart of aspiration—a moment of unconditional love.

I see clearly: my fear and antipathy toward those who exclude or diminish the people I care about is itself a form of othering. In reacting, I've mirrored what I resist. As I breathe and hold my own fear, I find—at least for a moment—the spaciousness to hold theirs as well.

Breathing in, I touch their fear.

It tastes the same as mine—the same bodily sensations, the same nervous system response. Only the object of fear is different. They fear what seems unfamiliar, what feels like a threat—just as I do. They voted with care, just as I did, based on the news and perspectives available to them, hoping it was the right choice. This recognition gives me solid ground to stand on when the rising tide of fear threatens to sweep me away in anxiety and outrage.

Breathing out, I smile, letting go of wrong perceptions of "us" and "them."

*Breathing in, my heart softens.*
*Breathing out, it fills with love.*
*I wish for them everything I most want for myself.*
*May they be well, may they be happy.*
*May we all enjoy the freedom of spiritual awakening.*
*May we all enjoy ease and tranquility.*

In these polarized times, I take heart in the stories of the Buddha's own trials. He had enemies. Some tried to fracture the Sangha; others tried to take his life. One story tells of an angry man who hurled insults at him. The Buddha remained calm, listening deeply. The man grew more agitated when he saw the Buddha was unmoved by his outburst. In exasperation, he demanded to know why. With kindness and equanimity, the Buddha replied: "If you give someone a gift and they refuse it, who does the gift belong to?"

The man scoffed. "To me, of course."

The Buddha said, "Just so. If I do not accept the gift of your abuse, it remains yours. Your unhappiness does not need to become my own."

Some friends express their care by posting the latest political outrage on social media. I appreciate their concern and their commitment to justice. At the same time, I know my peace and happiness are not separate from those on the other side. We are all in this together. Am I growing unity or division?

By now, we've discovered the futility of trying to change someone's mind. Expressing outrage often adds fuel to the flames of affliction. And yet, silence can feel like complicity. We all want to be heard, understood, and valued. I aspire to listen deeply.

Sometimes silence is complicity; other times, it is the sacred silence of one addict listening to another—without fixing, defending, or interrupting.

It may feel like agreement when we don't offer a rebuttal. But often, it is the gift of equanimity: being fully present with curiosity, interest, and a genuine desire to understand. When someone feels truly heard—even in disagreement—hearts touch, bridging the gulf in ways that words alone cannot. Sharing presence without attachment is a quiet joy.

Unconditional love is possible, at least for a breath or a moment. But like all formations, it is impermanent. Its seeds can be watered so it arises more often, its flower nourished to bloom a moment longer.

## The Gifts

The gifts of recovery are much more than abstinence, yet that's often how we measure success. Serenity, clarity, and freedom are harder to quantify. Focusing on time in recovery can lead to grasping and the mistaken belief that more is always better. For friends returning from relapse, it can deepen shame. Time is valuable. It marks our consistency and commitment. But how we live each moment—showing up with honesty, humility, and love—matters more.

Moments of awakening can arise suddenly and unexpectedly, in the meeting rooms and out in the world. Some people walk into their first meeting, hear the message, feel at home, and are instantly freed from the obsession to drink or use. But the awakening of the Twelfth Step is gradual, the result of working the previous eleven Steps. I did not "get struck" sober, but every bit of time and effort has been worth it.

In Buddhist scriptures we read about sudden and gradual enlightenment. In "The Fourteen Verses on Meditation," Thich Nhat Hanh writes:

> *Nirvana is non-attainment.*
> *Sudden or gradual enlightenment are not different.*
> *True realization is to live in freedom,*
> *right now, in this moment.*

The Buddha taught for forty-five years after his awakening beneath the bodhi tree. Did his understanding deepen over that time? Most assuredly. Shaped by his time and culture, he was initially unwilling to ordain women. When his foster mother and aunt requested ordination, he refused three times. His beloved disciple Ananda approached him and asked whether women had the same capacity for awakening as men. When the Buddha acknowledged that they did, Ananda gently suggested they be allowed to receive the same benefits of the Sangha. The Buddha remained teachable. His understanding continued to unfold.

There are still some Buddhist traditions that do not ordain women. It's a reminder that change is gradual and that deeply held views can endure, even within spiritual communities. We only see what we're ready to see. Insight ripens slowly. I've sat through Twelve-Step book studies for decades and still find lines that leap off the page with fresh meaning. The text hasn't changed; I have.

As Chögyam Trungpa Rinpoche emphasized in his lectures in the 1970s, everything is either poison or medicine—it depends on how you take it. For decades, I believed intoxicants were medicine, but they proved to be poison. In early recovery, I was proud of being a skilled thief; as my perspective changed, what once seemed like an asset was revealed as a shortcoming. As we grow, our understanding ripens. We see things differently.

Attachment to views is an obstacle to freedom. It's not easy to make use of hurt, grief, rejection, or even slanderous accusations, yet these can be gifts in disguise. The mess of our lives is the ground of liberation when we are resourced and trust the tools of transformation. This is the wisdom of the First Noble Truth: yesterday's bottom can become today's freedom.

There is a popular expression: "Shit happens." What we think of as shit can be composted and turned into fertilizer when we know how. With wisdom, we nourish the flowers, not the weeds. We know what we want to grow.

We are always practicing something. In every moment, we transmit our inner state.

While visiting Brother Pháp Hải in the Blue Mountains of Australia, we stopped in Blackheath for coffee after a cliffside meditation. As we approached the cafe, I noticed two elderly women having tea outside. The one facing us looked up, wide-eyed, and offered a shy smile. That's not unusual; walking alongside two robed monks with shaved heads tends to draw attention. We took a window seat indoors, and the same woman kept peeking at us. I took it as friendly curiosity and appreciated the warmth and openness of the locals.

As we were finishing our coffees, the woman approached Pháp Hải. "I'm sorry," she said gently. With his natural warmth and genuine interest, he asked, "Whatever for?" She glanced at me, then back at him. "My brother passed away recently," she said. "It's been a hard time." Pháp Hải gently took her hand in both of his, offering nothing but kind presence. She paused for a breath before adding, "When you walked up"—she paused again—"you looked so serene. It was like a refreshing breeze that cut through my sorrow."

I was gobsmacked. Her words were a lion's roar in the silence that followed. In that ordinary moment, as we walked in from the parking lot, Pháp Hải's presence, his very footsteps, eased her grief. No sermon. No advice. Just being.

When we embody our recovery, when we live our freedom, it is palpable. It liberates others. No words are needed. Thay could walk with such embodied peace that people I know were inspired to give up everything and enter upon the monastic path. The Buddha never declared himself awakened; his presence transmitted it with calm dignity. When children in the village first saw him, they exclaimed, "Buddha!"—the Awakened One. Our joy of living is a precious transmission, a gift infused with dignity and love.

## Riding the Waves of Deathlessness

After many years of committed practice and Sangha building, the community of Dharma Teachers in our tradition put my name forward to receive the Lamp of Wisdom. Without my knowledge, lay

Dharma Teachers and monastics wrote letters of support on my behalf, and I was invited to receive the Lamp. It was a great honor.

The Lamp of Wisdom has been handed down through generations of teachers since the time of the historical Buddha. It is not an arrival, but a threshold—a vow to keep practicing, to honor the lineage of ancestral teachers, to keep learning, and to grow in skillfulness. The trust of the community was humbling, and I vow to be worthy of it.

In the transmission ceremony, the recipient offers an insight gatha to the ancestral teachers. It expresses the fruit of our understanding and practice. If the ancestors accept it, the aspirant receives a transmission gatha in return. Leading up to the ceremony, I wrote many insight gathas: some simple, some poetic, some musical, and a few too wordy.

One was as spare as breath itself:

*Heart full,*
*no words needed.*
*Breathing in,*
*a smile is born.*

Others reached for deeper themes. The image of a lotus in the flames from Thay's cremation ceremony and the title of his wartime book, *Vietnam: Lotus in a Sea of Fire,* inspired a few gathas. Each touched the truth and were close to saying what was in my heart—but none were quite right.

When my beloved wife Betty and I traveled to Hawaii for a week to unplug from the noise of politics and enjoy our togetherness, I went scuba diving for the first time since recovering from valley fever. The water was murky, and I watched air bubbles rise slowly toward the surface, joining the open sky. That moment inspired the insight gatha I later offered:

*Bubbles of bodhicitta rise through the murky depths,*
*in the ocean of blues mmm a bird holds the sky.*

*Love warms the unloveable, the Dharma bell rings.*
*Ahhh a chrysanthemum blooms.*

Bodhicitta is the mind of unconditional love—the heartfelt wish that all beings be free from suffering. We swim in the conditioned reality of the historical dimension: an ocean of blues—sorrow, sickness, heartbreak, and loss. But when our nervous system is regulated and we are in harmony, we can hold this ocean of suffering in the spacious sky of liberation.

As we generate bubbles of love, they rise through the murky depths of the world and join the vast blue sky of nirvana—the image of a bird holding the sky. "Mmm" is the sound of humming, of Om, of shamatha—calm abiding. "Ahhh" is a sound of arrival and release.

The blooming chrysanthemum, Thay's favorite flower, is my teacher's continuation. During the procession to his cremation, cars and floats overflowed with chrysanthemums. The flower is Thay's smile, continued in me—and in us.

The "mmm" and "ahhh" came at the last moment, when I chose to sing and chant the gatha as a offering. I was nervous, but it was jazz—spontaneous and improvised. Fortunately, the ancestors dug it and accepted my gatha. Phew. They offered the following transmission gatha in return, which brought tears to my eyes:

*There is true joy in finding that waves*
*are made of the deep ocean water.*
*You ride on the waves of deathlessness*
*and bring fearlessness to the fearful.*

This gatha, inspired by my Dharma name, Chân Hỷ Hải—True Ocean of Joy—touches the depths of my aspiration, both in recovery and in all areas of my life: to bring fearlessness to the fearful. In times like these, non-fear may be the greatest gift we can offer.

When we touch the unlovable with the warmth of our love, in meditation and in Step work, we have become the living Dharma, the living program. The Dharma bell rings. The ancestors rejoice.

I am deeply grateful to have encountered the Buddha's teachings and the path of recovery. Many generations have passed without access to these teachings. To receive them, to live them, and now to share them is an immense privilege. It is an honor to be a lineage holder—empowered to transmit the Five Mindfulness Trainings, offer a lineage name to new friends, and share the Plum Village tradition.

It is also a great privilege to be a holder of our program, and to share the wisdom path of Twelve-Step awakening.

We are all teachers. May we each have the clarity to recognize what we transmit, the mindfulness to nurture our most precious aspirations, and the courage to walk the path—together.

Are you living right?

# ACKNOWLEDGMENTS

I offer deep gratitude to my parents, teachers, friends, and all who have supported my healing and transformation. Thank you.

To my sponsors, living and dead, who have walked with me on the path of recovery—listening and teaching with love and care, standing with me through good times and my darkest hours: Freddy Aquino, Hamilton (Ham) Morehead, Hank Magdaleno, and Bill Ryan.

To my recovery community, whose heart and indomitable resilience sustain me.

To Dan Howard, lifelong friend, writer, editor, brother in crime, and recovery companion, who has listened deeply, edited generously, and supported this book from its inception through its many iterations.

To Kevin Griffin, friend and brother on the path, whose encouragement and guidance have been invaluable in shaping this book, and whose prolific writing on Buddhist recovery helped plant the seed of this exploration decades ago.

To Matthew Friberg, friend, Dharma brother, and publisher, whose vision, interest, and steady encouragement sustained me as I found my way as a first-time author.

To Miranda Perrone, a friend and steadfast editor, whose insight and skillfulness have helped me refine my craft and improve the manuscript immensely.

To Karen Hilsberg and Alex Cline, dear friends who offered faith and love throughout the development of this book and the twisty road of life.

To the beta readers whose skillful comments and generous feedback have left their imprint on these pages.

To my dharma siblings in the 12-Step Zen and Open Heart Sanghas, whose practice and insight have so deeply nourished my own.

To John Chöpel Bruna, a wise teacher, friend, and fellow traveler on the path, whose embodied bodhicitta continues to inspire me.

To Jeff Zlotnik and Maggie Lee of the Dharma Bum Temple, for offering 12-Step Zen a home and a refuge for our community.

To Brother Pháp Lưu, Brother Pháp Dung, and Sister Đẳng Nghiêm, whose guidance and example have profoundly shaped both my living practice and this book.

To Dr. Peggy Rowe-Ward and Reverend Dr. Larry Ward of the Lotus Institute, in gratitude for your love, guidance, and inspiration.

To Brother Pháp Hải, who embodies the practice so beautifully, shares it so clearly, and cares so deeply—thank you for your wisdom, friendship, and support over the decades.

To Betty, my sweet wife, for your tender love, courage, and care—for walking this path with me. To Paola and Michelle, for welcoming me into your family and sharing your love so generously.

And to you, dear reader, thank you.

# THE TWELVE STEPS OF NARCOTICS ANONYMOUS

1. We admitted that we were powerless over our addiction, that our lives had become unmanageable.
2. We came to believe that a Power greater than ourselves could restore us to sanity.
3. We made a decision to turn our will and our lives over to the care of God as we understood Him.
4. We made a searching and fearless moral inventory of ourselves.
5. We admitted to God, to ourselves, and to another human being the exact nature of our wrongs.
6. We were entirely ready to have God remove all these defects of character.
7. We humbly asked Him to remove our shortcomings.
8. We made a list of all persons we had harmed, and became willing to make amends to them all.
9. We made direct amends to such people wherever possible, except when to do so would injure them or others.
10. We continued to take personal inventory and when we were wrong promptly admitted it.
11. We sought through prayer and meditation to improve our conscious contact with God as we understood Him, praying only for knowledge of His will for us and the power to carry that out.

12. Having had a spiritual awakening as a result of these steps, we tried to carry this message to addicts, and to practice these principles in all our affairs.

# THE THREE REFUGES*

*I take refuge in the Buddha,*
*the one who shows me the way in this life.*
*I take refuge in the Dharma,*
*the way of understanding and of love.*
*I take refuge in the Sangha,*
*the community that lives in harmony and awareness.*
*[BELL]*
*Dwelling in the refuge of Buddha,*
*I clearly see the path of light and beauty in the world.*
*Dwelling in the refuge of Dharma,*
*I learn to open many doors on the path of transformation.*
*Dwelling in the refuge of Sangha,*
*shining light that supports me, keeping my practice free of obstruction.*
*[BELL]*
*Taking refuge in the Buddha in myself,*
*I aspire to help all people recognize their own awakened nature,*
*realizing the mind of love.*
*Taking refuge in the Dharma in myself,*
*I aspire to help all people fully master the ways of practice*
*and walk together on the path of liberation.*
*Taking refuge in the Sangha in myself,*
*I aspire to help all people build fourfold communities,*
*to embrace all beings and support their transformation.*
*[BELL, BELL]*

---

* Thich Nhat Hanh, *Chanting from the Heart*, vol. 1, (Parallax Press, 2023), 108.

# THE FIVE MINDFULNESS TRAININGS*

Dear Sangha, this is the moment when we enjoy reciting the Five Mindfulness Trainings together. The Five Mindfulness Trainings represent the Buddhist vision for a global spirituality and ethic. They are a concrete expression of the Buddha's teachings on the Four Noble Truths and the Noble Eightfold Path, the path of right understanding and true love, leading to healing, transformation, and happiness for ourselves and for the world. To practice the Five Mindfulness Trainings is to cultivate the insight of interbeing, or Right View, which can remove all discrimination, intolerance, anger, fear, and despair. If we live according to the Five Mindfulness Trainings, we are already on the path of a bodhisattva. Knowing we are on that path, we are not lost in confusion about our life in the present or in fears about the future.

## Reverence For Life

Aware of the suffering caused by the destruction of life, I am committed to cultivating the insight of interbeing and compassion and learning ways to protect the lives of people, animals, plants, and minerals. I am determined not to kill, not to let others kill, and not to support any act of killing in the world, in my thinking, or in my way of life. Seeing that harmful actions arise from anger, fear, greed, and intolerance, which in turn come from dualistic and discriminative thinking, I will cultivate openness, nondiscrimination, and nonattachment to views in order to transform violence, fanaticism, and dogmatism in myself and in the world.

---

* Thich Nhat Hanh, *Chanting from the Heart*, vol. 2, (Parallax Press, 2023), 46–49.

## True Happiness

Aware of the suffering caused by exploitation, social injustice, stealing, and oppression, I am committed to practicing generosity in my thinking, speaking, and acting. I am determined not to steal and not to possess anything that should belong to others; and I will share my time, energy, and material resources with those who are in need. I will practice looking deeply to see that the happiness and suffering of others are not separate from my own happiness and suffering; that true happiness is not possible without understanding and compassion; and that running after wealth, fame, power and sensual pleasures can bring much suffering and despair. I am aware that happiness depends on my mental attitude and not on external conditions, and that I can live happily in the present moment simply by remembering that I already have more than enough conditions to be happy. I am committed to practicing Right Livelihood so that I can help reduce the suffering of living beings on earth and reverse the process of global warming.

## True Love

Aware of the suffering caused by sexual misconduct, I am committed to cultivating responsibility and learning ways to protect the safety and integrity of individuals, couples, families, and society. Knowing that sexual desire is not love, and that sexual activity motivated by craving always harms myself as well as others, I am determined not to engage in sexual relations without mutual consent, true love, and a deep, long-term commitment. I resolve to find spiritual support for the integrity of my relationship from family members, friends, and sangha with whom there is support and trust. I will do everything in my power to protect children from sexual abuse and to prevent couples and families from being broken by sexual misconduct. Seeing that body and mind are interrelated, I am committed to learning appropriate ways to take care of my sexual energy and to cultivating the four basic elements of true love—loving kindness, compassion, joy, and inclusiveness—for the greater happiness of myself and others. Recognizing the diversity of human experience, I am committed not to discriminate against any form of gender identity or sexual orientation. Practicing true love, we know that we will continue beautifully into the future.

## Loving Speech and Deep Listening

Aware of the suffering caused by unmindful speech and the inability to listen to others, I am committed to cultivating loving speech and compassionate listening in order to relieve suffering and to promote reconciliation and peace in myself and among other people, ethnic and religious groups, and nations. Knowing that words can create happiness or suffering, I am committed to speaking truthfully using words that inspire confidence, joy, and hope. When anger is manifesting in me, I am determined not to speak. I will practice mindful breathing and walking in order to recognize and to look deeply into my anger. I know that the roots of anger can be found in my wrong perceptions and lack of understanding of the suffering in myself and in the other person. I will speak and listen in a way that can help myself and the other person to transform suffering and see the way out of difficult situations. I am determined not to spread news that I do not know to be certain and not to utter words that can cause division or discord. I will practice Right Diligence to nourish my capacity for understanding, love, joy, and inclusiveness, and gradually transform anger, violence, and fear that lie deep in my consciousness.

## Nourishment and Healing

Aware of the suffering caused by unmindful consumption, I am committed to cultivating good health, both physical and mental, for myself, my family, and my society by practicing mindful eating, drinking, and consuming. I will practice looking deeply into how I consume the Four Kinds of Nutriments, namely, edible foods, sense impressions, volition, and consciousness. I am determined not to gamble, or to use alcohol, drugs, or any other products which contain toxins, such as certain websites, electronic games, TV programs, films, magazines, books, and conversations. I will practice coming back to the present moment to be in touch with the refreshing, healing and nourishing elements in me and around me, not letting regrets and sorrow drag me back into the past nor letting anxieties, fear, or craving pull me out of the present moment. I am determined not to try to cover up loneliness, anxiety, or other suffering by losing myself in consumption. I will contemplate interbeing and consume in a way that preserves peace, joy, and well-being in my body and consciousness, and in the collective body and consciousness of my family, my society and the earth.

# THE FIFTY-ONE MENTAL FORMATIONS

## Five Universals

contact
attention
feeling
perception
volition

## Eleven Wholesome

faith
inner shame (or "inner clarity of right and wrong")
shame before others (or "honoring the other")
absence of craving
absence of hatred
absence of ignorance
diligence, energy
tranquility, ease
vigilance, energy
equanimity
non-harming

## Six Primary Unwholesome

craving, covetousness
hatred
ignorance/confusion
arrogance
doubt, suspicion
misperception, wrong view

### Five Particulars

intention
determination
mindfulness
concentration
insight

### Ten Wholesome (added by Thích Nhat Hanh)

nonfear
absence of anxiety
stability, solidity
loving kindness
compassion
joy
humility
happiness
feverlessness
freedom/sovereignty

## TWENTY SECONDARY UNWHOLESOME

### Ten Minor Secondary Unwholesome

anger
resentment, enmity
concealment
maliciousness
jealousy
selfishness, parsimony
deceitful, fraud
guile
violent intent
pride

### Two Middle Secondary Unwholesome
lack of inner shame
lack of shame before others

### Eight Greater Secondary Unwholesome
restlessness
drowsiness
lack of faith, unbelief
laziness
negligence
forgetfulness
distraction
lack of discernment

### Four Indeterminate
regret, repentance
sleepiness
initial thought
sustained thought

# RESOURCES

If these teachings resonate, I hope you'll find your way to a community—a meeting, a sangha, or both. The path deepens in relationship.

- The Plum Village App: a goldmine of guided meditations, Dharma talks, and other precious resources
- Plumline.org: a worldwide Sangha listing for virtual and local Sanghas in the Plum Village tradition
- The Buddhist Recovery Network—Buddhistrecovery.org: a global meeting locator for Dharma-oriented recovery meetings and related resources
- 12-Step Zen—12stepzen.org: for online meetings with the author

# RECOMMENDED READING

Bruna, John. *The Wisdom of a Meaningful Life: The Essence of Mindfulness*. Central Recovery Press, 2016.

Chödrön, Pema. *The Pocket Pema Chödrön*. Shambhala, 2008.

Griffin, Kevin. *Sought Through Meditation: Exploring Step Eleven through the Lens of Dharma*. One Breath Books, 2024.

Hải, Brother Pháp. *The Eight Realizations of Great Beings: Essential Buddhist Wisdom for Waking Up to Who You Are*. Parallax Press, 2021.

Hải, Brother Pháp. *Nothing To It: Ten Ways to Be at Home with Yourself*. Parallax Press, 2015.

Jacobs-Stewart, Thérèse. *Mindfulness and the 12 Steps: Living Recovery in the Present Moment*. Hazelden Publishing, 2010.

Không, Sister Chân. *Learning True Love: Practicing Buddhism in a Time of War*. Parallax Press, 2007.

Levine, Stephen. *Guided Meditations, Explorations and Healing*. Anchor Books, 1991.

Levine, Stephen. *A Gradual Awakening*. Anchor Books, 1979.

Nhat Hanh, Thich. *Be Free Where You Are*. Parallax Press, 2002.

Nhat Hanh, Thich. *Breathe You Are Alive: Sutra on the Full Awareness of Breathing*. Parallax Press, 2008.

Nhat Hanh, Thich. *Call Me by My True Names: The Collected Poems of Thich Nhat Hanh*. Parallax Press, 2022.

Nhat Hanh, Thich. *Heart of the Buddha's Teachings*. Parallax Press, 2015.

Nhat Hanh, Thich. *No Death, No Fear: Comforting Wisdom for Life. Riverhead Books, 2003.*

Nhat Hanh, Thich. *No Mud, No Lotus: The Art of Transforming Suffering*. Parallax Press, 2014.

Nhat Hanh, Thich. *Present Moment, Wonderful Moment: Verses for Daily Living*. 3rd ed. Parallax Press, 2022.

Nhat Hanh, Thich. *Transformation and Healing: Discourse of the Four Establishments of Mindfulness.* Parallax Press, 2002.

Rowe-Ward, Peggy, and Larry Ward. *Love's Garden: A Guide to Mindful Relationships.* Parallax Press, 2008.

Ward, Larry. *Morning Night: Poems on Spirit, Race, and Nature.* Lotus Moss Press, 2025.

## ABOUT THE AUTHOR

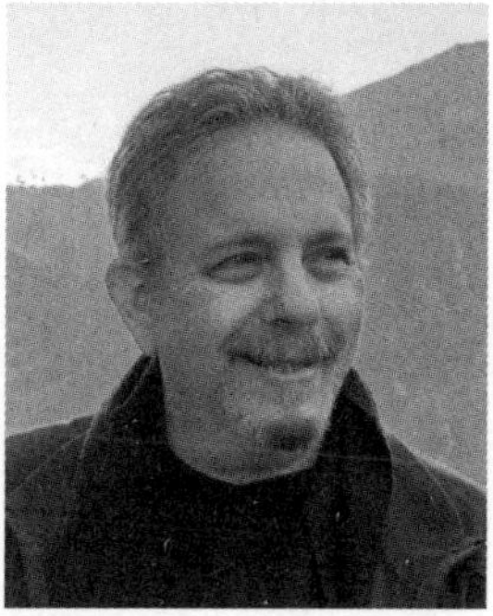

Peter Kuhn is a longtime practitioner in the Plum Village Zen tradition and a passionate advocate for healing through recovery and Dharma. After entering his first treatment program at age fourteen, he spent two decades in active addiction before beginning a path of spiritual transformation in 1986. Ordained by Thich Nhat Hanh in 2011 as "True Ocean of Joy," he cofounded True Freedom, a prison pen-pal program, and has led Twelve-Step Zen groups for more than a decade.

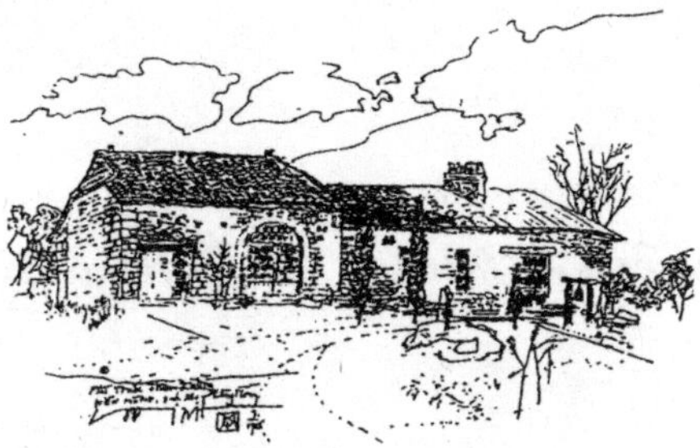

Monastics and visitors practice the art of mindful living in the tradition of Thich Nhat Hanh at our mindfulness practice centers around the world. To reach any of these communities, or for information about how individuals, couples, and families can join in a retreat, please contact:

**PLUM VILLAGE**
13 Martineau
33580 Dieulivol, France
plumvillage.org

**MAGNOLIA GROVE MONASTERY**
123 Towles Road
Batesville, MS 38606,
USA
magnoliagrovemonastery.org

**BLUE CLIFF MONASTERY**
3 Mindfulness Road
Pine Bush, NY 12566,
USA
bluecliffmonastery.org

**DEER PARK MONASTERY**
2499 Melru Lane
Escondido, CA 92026,
USA
deerparkmonastery.org

**EUROPEAN INSTITUTE OF APPLIED BUDDHISM**
Schaumburgweg 3
D-51545 Waldbröl, Germany
eiab.eu

**THAILAND PLUM VILLAGE**
Pong Ta Long, Pak Chong District
Nakhon Ratchasima
30130 Thailand
thaiplumvillage.org

**ASIAN INSTITUTE OF APPLIED BUDDHISM**
Ngong Ping
Lantau Island, Hong Kong
pvfhk.org

**LE MONASTÈRE DE A MAISON DE L'INSPIR**
8 Rue des Fans
77510 Villeneuve-sur-Bellot,
France
maisondelinspir.org

**HEALING SPRING MONASTERY**
2 Rue Pascal Jardin
77510 Verdelot, France
healingspringmonastery.org

**STREAM ENTERING MONASTERY**
221 Marias Lane
Beaufort, Victoria 3373, Australia
nhapluu.org

THICH NHAT HANH FOUNDATION

*planting seeds of Compassion*

THE Thich Nhat Hanh FOUNDATION works to continue the mindful teachings and practices of Zen Master Thich Nhat Hanh in order to foster peace and transform suffering in all people, animals, plants, and our planet. Through donations to the Foundation, thousands of generous supporters ensure the continuation of Thich Nhat Hanh's vision and help care for practice centers and monastics around the world. Your gifts help bring transformative practices to people who otherwise could not access them and support local mindfulness initiatives that ease suffering and cultivate joy.

By becoming a supporter, you join thousands of others committed to learning about, embodying, and sharing the life-changing practices of mindfulness, loving speech, deep listening, and compassion for oneself, each other, and the world.

For more information on how you can help spread Thich Nhat Hanh's teachings and practices globally, and to subscribe to our newsletters offering teachings, news, and information about retreats, please visit tnhf.org.

**Further Resources**

For information about our international community, visit: plumvillage.org

To find an online sangha, visit: plumline.org

For more practices and resources, download the Plum Village app: plumvillage.app